# The
# Language of
# Me

# The Language of Me

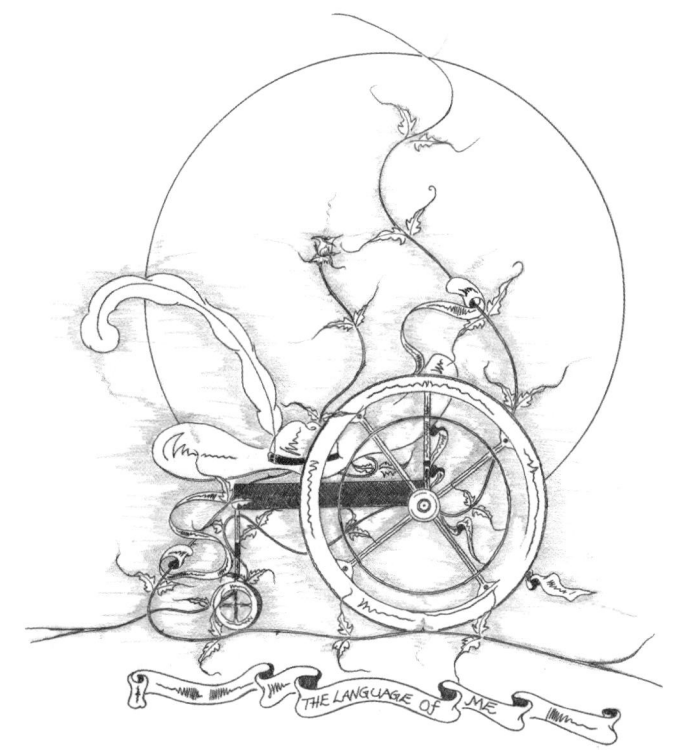

**MUSA E. ZULU**

UNIVERSITY OF KwaZulu-Natal PRESS

Published in 2004 by University of KwaZulu-Natal Press
Private Bag X01
Scottsville 3209
South Africa
Email: books@ukzn.ac.za
Website: www.ukznpress.co.za

© Musa E. Zulu 2004

Reprinted 2005, 2011

ISBN 1 86914 037 0

Editor: Elana Bregin
Concept and Cover Design: Flying Ant Designs
Layout: Alpha Typesetters cc, New Germany
Cover Photographs: Val Adamson

All rights reserved. No part of this publication may be reproduced or transmitted in any form or by any means, electronic or mechanical, including photocopying, recording or any information storage and retrieval system, without prior permission in writing from University of KwaZulu-Natal Press.

Printed and bound by Interpak Books, Pietermaritzburg

For my wife and my baby – my inspirations.

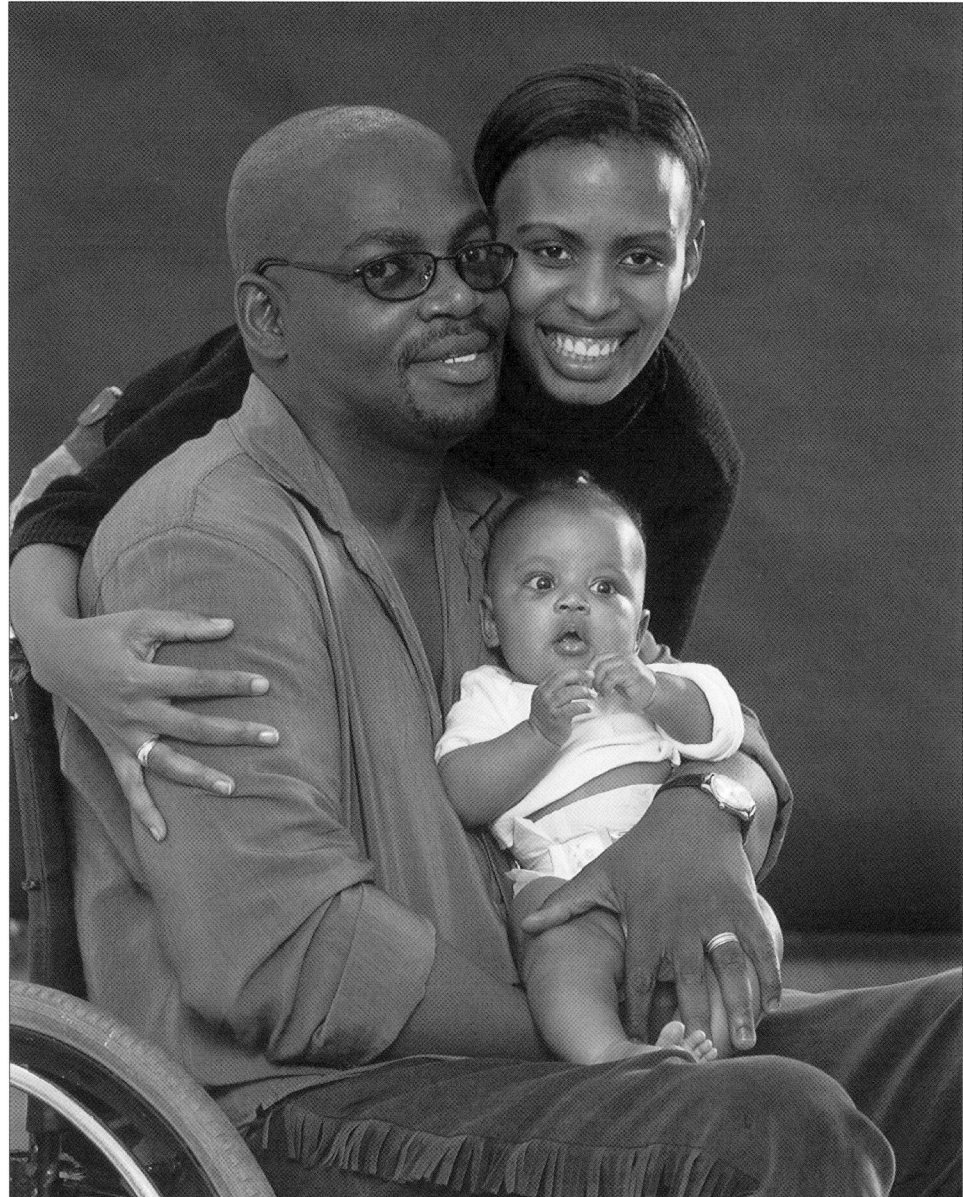

*Photo: Val Adamson*

*I would never wish to relive all my life!
Only a few very special and memorable moments,
for those define the evolution of my existence, the core of me,
and speak the true language of my emotions . . .
The Language of Me.*

# Change

Change . . .
A step in life
Once upon a time
We walked and danced
In the blink of an eye
All was changed

Pain . . .
A part of our lives
Yesterday you were here
We embraced and fell in love
Storms came sweeping
Clearing the plains

Sorrow . . .
We all go through it
The future stares in grief
As we rise and fall
Blown to the walls by the winds
Nothing is the same

Darkness . . .
Hatred invades our hearts and minds
Waging war against eternal peace
Drowning nature's smiles
Stealing light from the sky
The child paining with change

Death . . .
Fear grabs our souls
Tomorrow may not be here
A cold breeze blowing fallen leaves
Lonely tombstones with fading names
A mark of change and pain

Change and pain . . .
Moments that come for everyone
Yet you and I can heal
And escape from this prison
Steal away to a world of dreams
For a moment of peace and love

Yes, with love we can change the pain . . .

# Preface

## *Who is Disabled – Me or the World I Live in?*

Ever since the road accident in 1995 which left me paralysed and confined to a wheelchair, I have worked hard to enjoy my life, despite 'living with a disability', as they say. I was determined not to let my 'disability' keep me down and challenged myself to find a new life and, in the fullest sense of the word, live on. I have always been one to live my life to its ultimate potential and utilise the full range of my talents in the course of turning my dreams into reality. After the experience which changed my life, I felt compelled to write this book and share with others my 'dark night of the soul' – its highlights as well as its lowlights – and trace how the storms that I had gone through on my long journey back to the light had changed and reshaped me. In this way, I hoped to exorcise the ghost of 'disability' from the map of my life, and in its place hoist the flags of 'ability'.

I also, in 1995, had made a promise to my father that I would take the time to find myself through the hardships of paralysis and, in the end, write a story about my lessons. When an opportunity presents itself to me, it is in my nature to rise to the challenge. I always try to make the best of situations and turn them to my advantage, rather than allowing myself to be demoralised and have life's chances pass me by. The 20$^{th}$ of April was just such an opportunity, and I knew that the best way to survive the calamity was to find the good in it and make its challenges work for me rather than against me. I made a conscious resolution to learn from the event and keep its meaning alive for me – to celebrate its anniversaries, embrace the memories it reawakens, and hear its message ringing out loud and clear with the alarm-clock every morning; with the melodies of the church bells and wedding bells; and the songs of life and celebration that we gather together to share and sing in love.

Human existence is full of tragedy and trauma. Wars destroy families, societies and their cultures. Blue skies fill with the dust and smoke of destruction, and early dark engulfs the world. Everything that matters is destroyed as the Beast consumes the Beauty. Ghost towns ... fear ... it all seems so unreal. No one can predict what tomorrow will bring, or if there will be a tomorrow at all. Life is reduced to despair and tears ... prayers, hopes and wishes ... the pain of lost dreams and vanished loved ones ...

Yet after the war, humankind regroups, sharing the experiences of loss and embracing the light again. Peace revisits the world as the different races pull together in harmony, working to rebuild what has been destroyed. Fallen towers are re-erected, shattered glass is swept away, and the raging fires burn down to dying embers. Children play joyfully on open fields and lovers pace in slow motion, hand-in-hand beside the flowing streams. The evil of anger and hatred hides its menacing face behind shadows and tombstones. Hope, love and happiness are reclaimed and dreams are born again. The stories of life have many glorious endings, the texts of tragedy punctuated with accounts of miracles and amazing tales of happiness in the wake of sorrow.

It was my wish when I set out to write this book that after reading my story, a 'disabled' child, or a family with a member who is living with 'disability', might find new strength, might be inspired to embrace hope again and rise to the challenges of creating a better tomorrow for themselves and their loved ones. I wrote this book to tell a story of hope and to remind the world of the power of positive thinking. However, my story also points to the disabilities that I believe are constructed by society and which steal away from those affected, the opportunities for self-expression and a good life. These are what I refer to as social disabilities, imposed on us in various forms of discrimination: cultural stereotypes, prejudiced attitudes and the unfriendly infrastructure that 'able-bodied' societies construct in the name of mobility and commerce. Such 'disabling' factors need to be challenged head-on, for they are the discouraging winds that extinguish the vital, magical flame that burns inside our souls.

I feel truly blessed by life, given so much to be thankful for. I am alive, and I have learnt to appreciate fully what a gift that is. I am surrounded by people who love me and support me, and I've been given so many wonderful opportunities to exercise my talents and express the core 'music' that is me. I have more belief now in the beauty and purpose of life than ever before. But there are thousands of others who are a lot less fortunate, who are stuck away in the isolated rooms and solitary confinement of their disability, living lonely shadow lives of frustration and despair. It is my fervent wish to touch their lives with the magic of possibility. I believe very strongly that no matter what happens to us in life, we all have the capacity to succeed and be happy through the adversities. Give someone a chance to prove themselves, and you will be amazed at the wealth of talent and ability that reveals itself. When the burning flame of spirit is ignited, it can light up and transform any life, no matter what the circumstances.

This book is a record of my life between 1995 and 2001, the years of my journey through the light and shadow of disability. It is presented in two parts: the first tells the story of my 'Life After The Storm', and the second, I have called 'The Scrapbook Of My Soul'. This contains a selection of the sketches, poems and prose reflections I produced over the same period. All of these pieces trace my different emotional states through the many changes that I have been through and reflect different facets of the 'inner me'. My intention in presenting the book in this way is to show the world that 'disability' is not only a story to tell to others, but also a site of talents that deserve to be uncovered and exhibited. Many people do not believe that a person 'living with a disability' is capable of achieving 'the best'. I hope that this display of my 'diversity' as well as my 'difference' will help to change those stereotypes and give some insight into the dynamic and multi-faceted soul that resides in a disabled body.

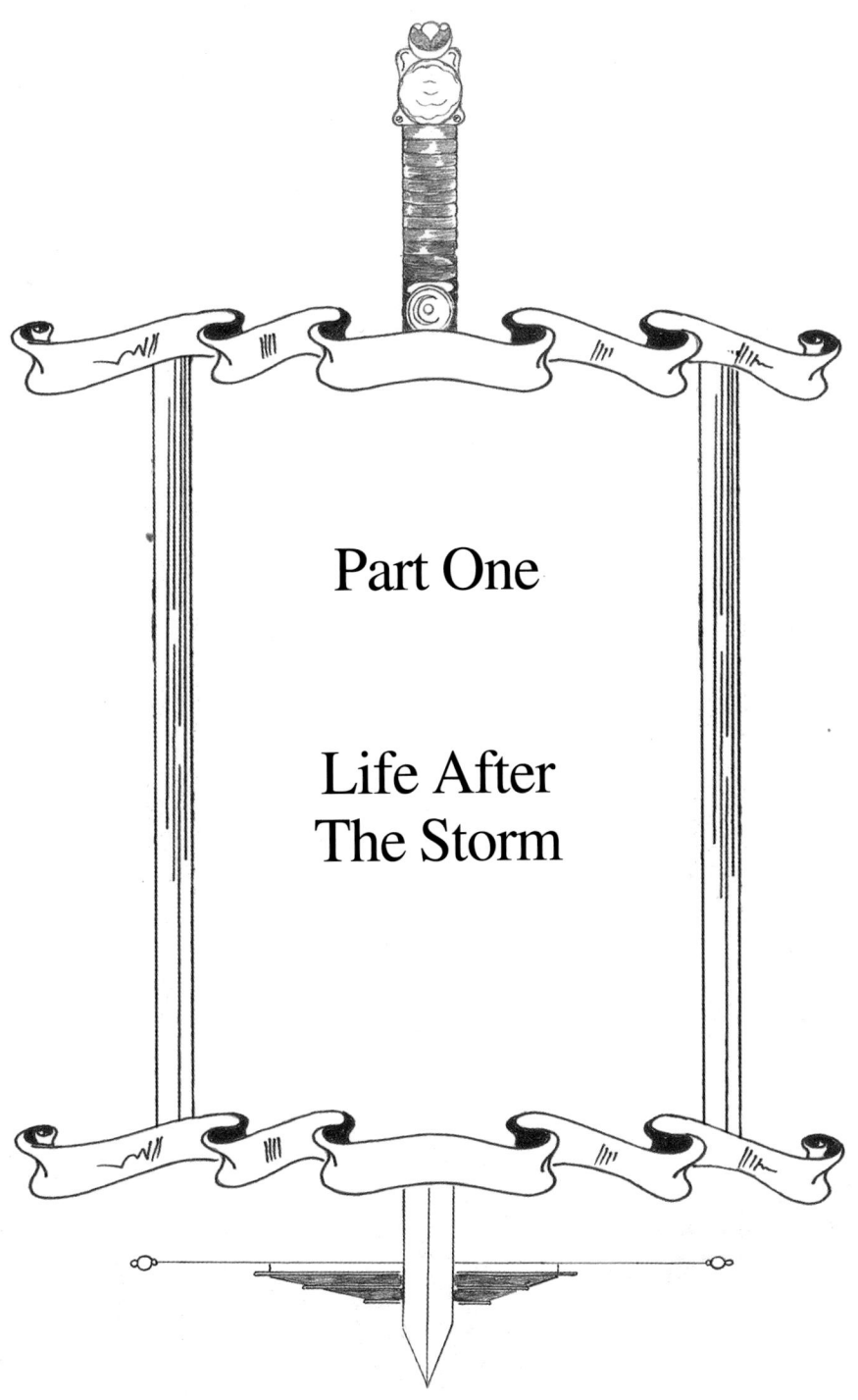

Part One

Life After
The Storm

# *On The 20<sup>th</sup> Of April . . .*

On the 20<sup>th</sup> of April it is an Anniversary
'Remembrance Day' – it says in my diary
A celebration and an examination of the changes
The story of a boy and a man on the pages

On the 20<sup>th</sup> of April I cried and I wept
Feeling the cold in the wind as I was swept
For walking these valleys was not just another act
It was a part of me and that was a fact!

On the 20<sup>th</sup> of April I reflect on a journey
That not only myself but others who are many
Travel and live through its fears and pains
Hoping for a home and love on these lonely plains

On the 20<sup>th</sup> of April to myself I made a promise
To cry, heal and move on in peaceful bliss
To battle with the fog that hums in crazy song
And find the clear skies that stretch along

On the 20<sup>th</sup> of April I assured my father and my brother
And I also said these words to my sister and my mother
That my world was beautiful and always will be
That with time I'd open my wings and fly like a bee

On the 20<sup>th</sup> of April I struck a deal
I made a wish and I wrote my will
To live my life, represent myself and be snappy
Today I am alive and my story is happy

Every year on that day I am called to account
For it is on that day that I come to find myself
And remember that it is still ME and always will be
On the 20<sup>th</sup> of April . . .

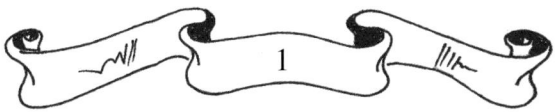

It was raining hard that evening. I still remember those heavy April rains. It was about 9.30 p.m. and I was travelling north along Umbilo Road – for what reason I can't say. The last thing I clearly recall is driving into Quentin's BP Petrol Station – whether for petrol, to pick up a cooldrink or some chewing gum, or some other purpose, I'm not sure; since I knew the attendants there, it might have been that I just wanted to share a joke with the boys. I don't remember actually buying anything or leaving the petrol station. I have tried many times to piece together what happened along Umbilo Road that evening, but there is very little that I have managed to retrieve from my memory. Whenever I reflect on those final moments, I only see flashes of bleak scenes that light up and dim away in my mind: drops of hard rain on the windscreen . . . cold showers of drizzle on my face . . . bright flashing lights. I faintly remember the commotion – someone pulling me out of the wreck, the sound of my own cries ringing inside my head. That's all. The rest is a blank. A witness from a nearby block of flats testified that she heard two loud bangs, the first like the sound of two cars colliding, then a second impact. She also claims to have seen another car in the middle of the road, but whether that car was involved in the accident, or belonged to a passerby who had stopped to help, no one can say. I have no memory of a collision, or of my car spinning out of control to smash against the brick wall in Umbilo Road; I can't recall the pain of impact, being admitted to hospital, the first days in ICU or anything else about the drama. For the next four days after the crash there was complete quiet and darkness all around me. Just quiet, not even a dream.

    Then snap – I woke up! I looked around and knew instantly where I was. I could tell I was in a hospital ward by the smells – the slight odour of blood, the nauseating stench of medication and chemicals that hovered in the air of the cold room. The cold is what stands out in my memory. It was a cold not just of temperature, but of the whole environment – a chill that permeated to the core of me. I was in a room full of inert white bodies, stacked in rows of beds against the walls. I felt like I was in a Sci-Fi movie. It was early in the morning when I surfaced, around 4 a.m. and still dark. There was no one around to comfort me or answer my questions. I discovered there was a drip attached to my arm and I remember the panic I felt as I tried to lift my head but could not. Every attempt sent me spinning into blackness. The effort of moving was akin to trying to lift up the whole galaxy. It was clear that something terrible had happened to me, but what it was I could not tell. It was hard to think straight. I was still very woozy from the sedatives, drifting in and out of consciousness and reality. I felt confused, helpless, terrified and yearned for the morning light, for people, explanations, answers . . .

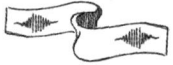

The sanctity of family is a critical factor in the shaping of one's personality and growth. I come from a big extended family, one of six siblings – the third-born after my twin sisters, Babongile and Bongiwe. I also have a younger brother, Thabani, who comes directly after me, followed by two small sisters, Khetiwe and Thulisile. Our house has always been full of children, not just the off-spring of my mother's womb, but those of family relatives: small and grown-up, quiet and loud-spoken, lean and fat, naughty and 'every-proud-parent's-dream'. Because of the 'population explosion' at home, my world has always been made up of 'we' and 'us'. I cannot recall a time in my life when it was ever just 'me'. My background created my personality. Because I grew up in a crowd, my thoughts have always been shared. Looking back on the history of my life, I am struck by my good fortune in having the strong support networks that I have had. Whatever the experience, however challenging the road, I was never alone through any of it. There was always someone to share in the events and travel the journey with me – to stand by me, guide and advise me. I enjoy keeping close company with those who are dear to me, talking away for hours with them, sometimes deep into the night. I am simply not one for keeping my own company. The Zodiac decreed that I should be a Sagittarius, and I am the classic extrovert, comfortable in the company of others, talkative and free with my affection. I love the limelight and am never happier than when in the centre of a crowd.

I grew up closely connected with my large army of 'brothers' and 'sisters'. Back in the late 70s and early 80s, when we were still a very young crowd, all of us little ones went to church together, following each other in a line, hand-in-hand along the road, like baby elephants holding onto each other's tails. I don't know if this tendency was born out of fear that one of us would be suddenly snatched away or was simply a sign of our close bonding. As a family, we always had our favourite old-time stories to refer back to, remembering the standard jokes and laughing like they had just been told for the first time. We woke up together and fell asleep together, talking away nineteen to the dozen and passing coded notes to the 'trusted buddies' among us, while evading those we perceived to be the 'spies' in the ranks, or 'mother's pets'. These were the ones outside of the 'naughty' group – those whom our mother knew could always be relied on 'to tell' if an iron or a window mysteriously got broken. Like every crowd, extended families have their internal divisions, and ours was no exception. We fought at times, but on the whole we remained good friends and leaned on each other through the trying times. Together, we spent long nights concocting a golden future for ourselves, where we would live out our ambitious dreams and progress to even greater things. What we dreamed of most was shining in a crowd, winning the adoration of a multitude of fans. We fantasised about being musicians, or stand-up comedians – even generals in the army, for this would give us the chance to wear a uniform and command others. Our parents taught us to share everything, not only among ourselves, but also with others less fortunate than we were. Ours was one of the emerging black middle-class families that became evident in the townships during the early 80s. We lived in a bigger house than the average township dweller, went to better schools, and were advantaged by our better education. Yet we never thought of ourselves as being 'a cut above' the rest. Everything we had, including the special tutoring my father conducted for us, was freely shared with others in the neighbourhood. From an early age, it was instilled in me to extend the same royal treatment to everyone who enters my home, regardless of who they are; to welcome them as friends and reserve a warm space at the table of my heart for strangers as well as those well-known to me. This is a philosophy that has won me many enduring friendships throughout my life.

On weekends, tennis was the big thing in our family. All of us would pile into my father's old Peugeot 404 and head off to the courts in Umlazi D Section, where the community would congregate. Regular tournaments were held there, attended by players from the adjoining Coloured and Indian communities. All of this changed in the 80s, with the institution of the Tricameral parliament, which realigned Coloureds, Indians and whites on the same side of the political fence and left blacks out in the cold. But up until that time, Umlazi, like the other townships, was a thriving centre of interactive activity, and on a weekend the tennis courts were the place to be. Those of us who could not fit into the family Peugeot would try to squeeze into one or other of my father's friends' cars. If you were unlucky enough not to get a lift, you were forced to stay at home, haunted by the walls and the loud quiet. We were not used to the experience of being alone. On one occasion, when my sister Babongile was left behind, we returned to find music blaring from the house, loud enough to lift the roof off, and Babongile looking very forlorn: 'It's very quiet here,' she complained, when asked the reason for her sad face.

We children did everything together. We all went to the same schools and had virtually the same friends. The nights were always abuzz with activity – play, song, dance ... casino, Monopoly, cowboys, toys ... friends. Later, in 1982, when we moved into a bigger house in the township, my father regularly gathered us all together, along with the children from neighbouring households, to give us extra lessons in English and writing. He introduced innovative ways of making the lessons easier – using word-games such as Scrabble, stories from *Reader's Digest*, and essay-writing assignments. Every outing to town – to the beachfront, Mini-Town, the countryside or Lion Park – was followed by an essay assignment which we submitted to my parents for reading and language corrections. We were encouraged to speak and write not only in English but also in Zulu. My father's emphasis with language was always on good style, creativity and clarity of meaning. My mother still has some of those old scripts locked away in a safety box, with all their mistakes and hilarious misunderstandings.

My father, Paulus Mzomuhle Zulu, was a very well-known and respected personality in our community. He was one of the first black academics to hold a lectureship at the University of Natal, in the Department of Social Science. What characterises him best in the eyes of those who know him is his dedication to breaking down barriers through promoting the culture of respect, and his gift for making people – friends and strangers alike – feel valued and loved. Education has always been my father's crusade. He understood the importance of giving his children a headstart in life through good schooling and a good command of language. This ideal extended to the children of our township in general. In the early 80s, together with his close friends, he started running a Saturday school. They went on to form SAPSWA – South African Black Worker's Association – making it their personal mission to improve literacy levels in the township and develop previously disadvantaged communities. I remember as a young boy the many weekend trips to my father's University office, where he loved to take us. He would give us some of his books to read to keep us busy while he completed his tasks and on our way back home, would quiz us about what we'd read, always happy when we answered correctly. I grew up wanting to be like him and loved listening to him when he lectured his students.

My mother, Nkosinathi Zulu, is someone who stands tall in any crowd. She has a very commanding presence, which comes from being the first-born in her family. She used to be a tutor at the Nursing School at McCord Hospital in Durban and is a natural teacher, with many lessons of wisdom to impart. It was my mother who taught me my love of beauty and to appreciate the gentler pleasures of life. I believe that I have inherited a big part of my personality, interests and hobbies from her. She is very creative in a hands-on way, as opposed to my father, who is creative with his head. She also draws well and is a good storyteller, spicing her tales with words aimed to stimulate the imagination of the listener. She loves looking beautiful, and holds the philosophy that if you are confident about your appearance, you will be more able to uncover the beauty and peace of mind that resides in the depths of the soul.

I love my family. They are my unit, my foundation and my strength. To me, the family is the cornerstone of a community, a society and the world. Family relations are what prepare us for the outside world – for 'the other' that we will encounter there. It's through family that we first come to know what is right and wrong, what can be achieved and by what means, and how to live through both joy and pain. This is what my family has taught me – that life can be beautiful and rich to those who work hard to earn its fruit; but that life can also be hard, and that one day everything falls to pieces and has to be picked up and rebuilt; that you have to allow for the change of those moments, and accept that there will be tears as well as laughter embodied in them. While there is a need to keep tomorrow in sight and bank for it, it is important to live as fully as you can today, for there may not be any tomorrow. It is also through my family that I have come to appreciate the importance and power of the 'Brotherhood', and to develop my respect, love and admiration for the 'Sisterhood'. It is because of the way my own sisters have conducted themselves, with dignity, humility and courage, that I have learnt to value those qualities in other women and approach them from that informed perspective.

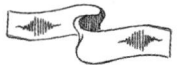

'No, you won't be able to walk again. The injuries you sustained are simply too serious for me to be able to offer any positive medical prognosis. You fractured your left clavicle, two of your floating ribs and also two vertebrae, T4 and T7. The impact created a whiplash effect which resulted in your sustaining an oedema down your spine at T6 level, and this caused instant paralysis. I'm sorry . . .'

The doctor went on speaking, in his unemotional, matter-of-fact voice. He was saying things about motor neurons . . . swollen nerves . . . MRI scanning . . . I heard the word 'wheelchair'. It all made very little sense to me – mere doctor's bullshit jargon. Every word he spoke confused and irritated me more, especially when he hinted that I might have to spend a few months in hospital. 'No ways!' was my instant reaction. I almost told him right there and then what to do with his diagnosis, but was deterred by the presence of my parents and the other elders, who were all gathered around my bed, looking very serious at the pronouncements. The mood was sombre and all the faces were wearing similar expressions, as if they were in pain – with the exception of the talkative doctor, who kept flashing his silly smiles, trying his level best to reassure everyone. I just lay there and listened, wishing he and his staff would hurry up and finish their business and leave – and take everyone else with them, so that I could be left in peace to sleep. That day went by like a lightning flash – the fastest day of my life. Many faces showed up at my bedside – family, friends, colleagues, strangers; my girlfriend was among them. But I was too tired and weak to give a damn about anything or keep tabs on who was there. Everyone was still going on about rehabilitation programmes and 'suitable institutions' when I went back to sleep . . .

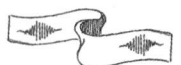

I received almost all of my school education in overcrowded township schools, with the exception of Sub-Standard A (equivalent to Class 1), which I did in a rural school in Ixopo, where my father's family still stays. This was back in 1977, when I was just six years old, and I have very little recollection of those early years. In 1978, we moved to Umlazi Township in Durban, where I continued my education until I matriculated eleven years later in 1988. During my primary school days, the boys called me 'D-Man'. I acquired this nickname after we had been watching a film at primary school called 'Mighty Man'. I am reminded by old friends that after the movie, I walked out of the room boasting: 'Mighty Man may be strong but I'm still "The Man".' Believe me, in our neighbourhood, I *was*

'The Man'. Because of the advantages my background gave me, in the form of privileged access to TV, books and other sources of knowledge, I was often one step ahead of everybody else. I was always the one with the big dreams and the confidence to believe in them. My natural leadership qualities allowed me to capitalise on my family's prominent status and live up to my own aspirations. D-Man remained my nickname all the way through primary school.

While in primary school, I joined the Boy Scouts and enjoyed going on camps with them to experience the wild outdoors and be with the boys. I couldn't wait for Thursdays, because that was the day our Scout troop assembled on the field for drill. This was show time; everybody, including the girls, would gather to watch the spectacle as we passed by in salute. Thursday was also 'interaction day', when the boys competed in activities such as making fires and vied among themselves to see who was the fastest in hoisting the flag and tying reef-knots. I loved the outdoor camps, which were held twice a quarter and always involved long walks into neighbouring rural areas, crossing rivers and climbing mountains. It was a liberating experience to be in such close contact with nature and I still remember the freedom and stimulation of those walks.

I was an extrovert even in those early days and my outgoing nature won me a lot of friends at school and in the township. Before I knew it, my wisecracking talk, together with a few hard-won Michael Jackson 'moonwalk' steps, had broadcast my fame to other neighbouring and distant townships. I was in great demand as an entertainer, called on to 'strut my stuff' at weddings, inter-school competitions, sportsdays and the like. Michael Jackson was my role model and I became adept at performing my breakdancing moves to his 'Thriller' songs; to the crowds, I *was* Michael Jackson. Fame brought its own problems, however, and it wasn't long before trouble started knocking insistently at my door. At school, I was a disruptive presence. My success with the crowds went to my head, and between my wisecracking in class and the noisy gatherings I attracted around me, I antagonised a lot of teachers. When the bell rang to signal the end of break, I would simply ignore it and continue dancing, with the result that the watching crowds would be too slow to disperse to their classes. I interacted with the headmaster's cane so frequently that it became my bosom buddy – the same was true at home. The numerous after-school requests I received to perform meant that I came home later and later, which also earned me my share of hidings.

I went AWOL from school a lot. I would do anything to get out of class; to me, chatting to friends was much more exciting than listening to the tie-and-suit-clad teachers who taught me. I found them far too formal and boring for my taste. Needless to say, my school performance took a dive and by my second year of high school, things had got totally out of hand. In July 1985, in the middle of the school term, my father decided to transfer me from my current school (where he quite rightly felt that I was drifting far astray) to the more reputable institution where my big sisters were studying and applying their minds much more successfully towards their education. I remember the discomfort of that first day. I was a stranger in a strange crowd who did not know anything about me or the world of fame I hailed from. I had no one to gossip with or pass secret notes to.

This sent my world tumbling down the drains of alienation and distanced me from my beloved crowds. My nickname, 'D-Man', was undone and Musa, my Zulu name, resurfaced. However, I would not say that this change had any lasting impact on my wild ways. I still skipped classes if I could, the difference being that at least now I got to devote a few more minutes to the piles of textbooks on the shelves, with the result that my school performance improved.

I had a natural aptitude for languages (with the exception of Afrikaans) and I also fared well in Agriculture and Biology. But I struggled with Physical Science and performed dismally in Mathematics. I never acquired a fondness for school. To my free spirit and happy-go-lucky nature, the early morning start and rigid rule systems were always a nightmare. While others were deep in their books during the afternoon study period, I would be watching Eddie Murphy in a movie theatre. When they were burning the midnight oil at their studies, I was out 'hunting' in the night. This was a time when members of the opposite sex were beginning to inscribe their various dots on the map of my life. One of the fringe benefits of my 'fame' was the way it brought females flocking into my orbit, all of them eager to be associated with 'Michael Jackson'. I was far from being one of the bright academic stars at school, but I featured prominently in 'The Noisemaker's Register' and was a known regular in 'The Lover's Pages'. I was not one for following rules, and this brought me into frequent conflict with 'the bureaucracy'. To me, prefects were sell-outs who enjoyed privileged attention from the staff and were 'every mother's dream' (never a good recommendation in my eyes). Throughout my school career, authority and I did not see eye to eye, and our confrontations always ended with my name in somebody's black book and yet another session with my 'bosom buddy'. As much as the teachers hoped that the corporal punishment they imposed would help to banish my rebel's streak, the scars they left on my butt to me represented just another mark in my defiance crusade. I was living my life the way I wanted it, maturing and growing with all my diverse experiences. Because of the range of activities that I had access to and the opportunities that I created for myself, my worldview was much wider than that of my little brother or my less adventurous peers, who lived more sheltered lives. My scouting activities took me out of the rigid and over-developed environs of the township and allowed me to connect with the outdoor world that I loved. My performances in front of a crowd gave me a lot of standing and status and the confidence to capitalise on it. I had the opportunity to interact with different sets of people and broaden not just my social skills, but my understanding of life. In general, I had a good childhood and even though I broke a couple of golden rules along the path, I learnt with every step I took. Those were 'the golden glory days' of my growing life. I was too young to be directly affected by the political turmoil that engulfed the townships in the 80s, and was to some extent sheltered from it by my family's position. I lived in my own world of fantasy, wrapped up in my self-absorbed dreams and ambitions; a carefree young boy, surfing the waves of the times.

## *Crescendo*

Angels descend from the skies
A bolt of lightning cracks the clouds
Violins greet the drums with cries
The Universe trembles as the stairway lands
And the Earth welcomes the heavens

Desperation, need – all the human feelings
The musician knows his lines
How could it be in this life
That an hour can be so dark?
Love can only be once found

Guitar strings trickled in a strum
Shelter, pleasure and loneliness
There he goes again, to the sky he vaults
Horns, violins, pianos and drums
The verse gives way to the chorus

Lamenting and reminiscing
I don't want no explanation
The thoughts shatter my mind
Only the heart knows what is now
And what could never be

Endless questions – is love forever?
Emptiness for the loveless, pain
Dreams of the lonely, despair
The need to be held and loved
Crescendo, voices conjure the spirits!

Mountains explode in volcanic eruption
The dragon soars from the ground – earthquakes
The conductor on the wings, pointing the charge
His fingers weaving the melody, waterfalls
No reasons can change what's gone . . .

Darkness slowly drifts from the sun
As the lullaby softly fades in pain
Rivers and streams dry up in realisation
And voices are drowned in the symphony
As the matador delivers the snorting bull . . .

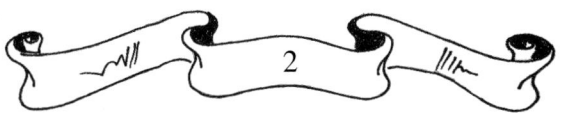

I grew up in a family that loves music: my father with his Beethoven and Handel, Johann Sebastian Bach and Franz Joseph Haydn, Mendelssohn, Mozart and many others – violins, cellos, horns and drums crashing and climbing in wonderful crescendos. My mother with her Country Music: Dolly Parton and Kenny Rogers – 'Islands in the Stream, that is what we are' – the legends of the countryside and cowboys. My Uncle Qhawe and his guitar; his favourite composition: *'Ngiyahamba ngiy' emazweni,* I am leaving to a world far away' – strings like liquid trickled in a strum. He would play and croon, lost in the melody of his own creation: *'Ngiyahamba ngiy'emazweni maye!'* Then that traditional uMbhaqanga rap. Everyone in the house, including his dangling wooden dolls, exploding into a sudden energy of 'jive and dance', enjoying the beat of the musical stampede. *'Khalaj!'* – the exclamation, as he pulls up his puppet dolls into a karate act symbolising a fight between two lovers about to part ways. His audience would roar. Then, the quietening mood as the sun sets and the guitarist remembers his sorrows. He reminisces, painting with his words the sights and heights of those evaporated glory days when the love was still burning hot – *'Ngiyahamba,* I am leaving'; now it's all gone. With his shoulders sagged to portray the pains of a jilted lover, my uncle the showman would fade away with his song into the shadows of the distant horizon. It was an amazing display of feeling and emotion, theatre in its most spontaneous form. I grew up in a homestead where it was not a shame to erupt into loud song inside the confining walls of a lavatory. We sang to the beat of pain and pleasure – life to us was a song worth singing!

I inherited the family love for music. I grew up listening and singing along to a whole range of sounds – Pop, Rock 'n Roll; iS'cathamiya – Dr Mshengu Shabalala and the legendary Black Mambazo; Heavy Metal, from Black Sabbath to Ronnie James Dio and Iron Maiden. I pounded my fist to the bass sounds of 'The Last in Line', head-banged to the 'Seventh Son of The Seventh Son' and 'Jumped' to my favourite Van Halen. These were the Monsters of Rock, and I 'moshed in the pit' of their pounding sounds for many years. I still have a denim jacket adorned with drawings and the badges of various heavy metal bands. In the words of Judas Priest, 'I'm a Rocker', and no one can take that away! One of my favourite musicians was Canadian-born David Foster – producer, song-writer and singer. With his 'classic rock' style he combined the best of two streams of musical orientation, tailoring his hits to suit the preferences of my own 'classics-illiterate' hard rock generation, while at the same time honouring the old classical gems so

...usic lovers like my father. I had great respect for his talents and spent ...l hours immersed in the musical Nirvana of his various 'Love ...other masterpieces.

...t hours listening to Soul ballads, while scribbling 'charming notes' ... 'sweethearts' who came and went in my life; Jazz and the Blues – ... Gary Moore – more than anything I love the sounds of a well-... guitar. I remember those 'crazy nights' as a growing boy picking up the household broom and 'raving havoc' with it to the sounds of the legendary Stevie Ray Vaughan. It's said that only the good die young – and that guy could play! I had posters of guitarists and their polished guitars all over my bedroom walls. Today, I still keep an acoustic guitar in my bedroom – a sexy work of art that is lovely to touch and a pleasure to strum. It goes without saying that in the course of my musical explorations, I also did not neglect to investigate the melodies of the 'Holy Herb' – Reggae, the protest cry of the oppressed; Bob Marley and Peter Tosh . . . 'Legalise It!' became my personal slogan too.

As a young boy I was always fascinated by the power that musicians have over people – the packed stadiums and the screaming fans, the pin-up pictures in numerous popular magazines and the gossip about their private lives that was exposed for public consumption. A people's person myself, I was inspired by the sight of the constant crowds that always surrounded the musicians. I marvelled at their stretch limousines and their sleek Harley Davidson motorbikes. I loved the way they dressed and the deference they received at press conferences – their skill in handling questions and the whole lifestyle of privilege and command that went with their fame.

At home, we were encouraged to listen to and read music and were pointed to 'the message' as the treasure to hunt for in the songs. My father believed that in this way we would improve our language skills. In 1987 my parents bought us a piano and my younger brother Thabani spent hours playing Richard Clayderman's tunes. Friends and members of our church choir would drop by to practise their gospel songs, and the house would explode with the off-key shrieks of voices battling to find the high notes. I walked the 5 kms to school with earphones pounding my soul with sweet sounds. Music was and still is so much a part of my life that I cannot envisage an existence without it. Songs are the heartbeat of my world, the background pulse to which I move and draw breath, guide my pencil and steer my car. Their lyrics are what conjure the memories of my past and the dreams of my future.

The poetry of music, and the music of poetry; to me, these are the vehicles for the deepest emotions that human nature can ever express. It is with the music and poetry of our souls that we communicate our pain, hopes and desires . . . our need to love and be loved . . . that inner quest to understand and be understood . . . and the wish to find a home and a place to belong. Music is the first language, the poetry of life expressed in the harmonies of God.

I have often wondered what my life would have been like had God given me the gift to create the scenes and sweet melodies of music. But since that was not the talent that God gave me, it was to poetry and writing that I turned to express the passions of my soul. My first experiments with the music of words started fairly early in my life. In my mid-teens, I enrolled at Vukuzakhe High School in Umlazi to do my Standard Nine. It was here that I began to exercise my discursive skills and participate in the debates and classroom discussions that were encouraged at Vukuzakhe as a means of fostering more active student involvement. I participated in virtually all the debates and student discussions during my two-year sojourn at that school and had the honour to represent the school in various inter-school symposiums.

I enjoyed my Vukuzakhe days and was happy to be at a school where a student's potential was actively encouraged and allowed to grow. My talent for attracting a reputation blossomed again – this time, it was as a school cartoonist and promising artist. I enjoyed drawing and loved to accompany my sketches with a few lines of prose or poetry – sometimes funny, sometimes straight, with an inspirational message. During this time I also featured quite prominently in the school stage plays, and together with four of my friends, 'topped the charts' in music competitions. 'The Gospel Train is coming, I hear it just at hand' was one of our favourites. All of this was laying the groundwork for the days to come, giving me the performance and rhetorical skills I would need to make my mark on audiences in my ordained career of the future – as a motivational speaker and campaigner for disabled rights. But, of course, I didn't know it then. All I knew was that I enjoyed standing up to speak in front of an audience. It was there, 'out in front', that I could exercise my mind and share my feelings with others. My early successes during my 'Michael Jackson' dancing days had given me the confidence to know I could hold the attention of a crowd. Those early days had also made me aware that I had the ability to touch hearts and minds with my words and leave a lasting impression. I never missed an opportunity to speak. My success with spoken language and the pleasure it gave me to 'toy' with words in front of an audience encouraged me to explore the art of the written word.

It started with 'lipstick letters', penned to the classroom 'queens' of the time, and soon became a hobby – to pick up a pen and capture that passing thought in ink. I found a wonderful freedom in these moments, soaring with each poetic word and creative line. I was dying to produce a 'real' poem, and started borrowing lines from my favourite songs, recombining them to create my own messages and meanings. I yearned for my own authentic spark of creation, to be able to put down my thoughts in a 'language' of words and style that was all mine. When I finally found that spark there was no holding back. The lines seemed to explode onto the page without conscious direction from me. The first poem I wrote in 1987 was called 'Fly Free Butterfly, Fly'. It was an expression of my own inner wish for freedom, a word painting of uninterrupted beauty. When the 'butterfly' was born and escaped into flight, I felt like a bird in the sky – cutting through the air in a dance of unrestrained ecstacy.

I read the poem out to the entire school during one of the School Literature Days. My principal, who had come to label me 'a notorious rebel', quickly responded by saying he would 'tolerate no butterflies' in his school. This earned me the nickname 'Butterfly' among my peers, which stuck with me for the rest of my duration at Vukuzakhe. In fact, my principal's objection was misplaced. Contrary to his interpretation, the poem was not a subversive expression of my opposition to the schooling system under which I studied, or even to the larger political system that excluded my people from political and economic participation. It represented a more universal desire for nature to be allowed to come into its own and flaunt its spectacular beauty without restriction. In spite of my principal's reaction, I was elated by my success that day. I knew I had achieved a longheld dream – to use poetic language to express the message in me and find a way to translate 'talk' into the written word.

That same day, Mr Majola, my English teacher of the time, approached me and praised my achievement. He listened attentively as I explained to him the meaning behind the lines. He was very appreciative of the poem itself, as well as of the fact that one of his students was showing signs of a love for poetry – his ultimate passion. He pointed out the ways in which I could improve the structure of my poem through better shaping of the lines and clearer portrayal of my ideas.

I looked up to Mr Majola and spent a lot of time talking my ideas through with him and reading to him to improve my language and command of words. His emphasis was always on balance and clarity of expression, and the careful selection of words for maximum effect. He was an excellent speaker of the 'white-man's-tongue' and spent most of his free time reading his Bible, Shakespeare, Greek philosophy and poems by the classical poets. A devoted member of the Roman Catholic Church and an acclaimed composer, producer and conductor of choral songs, he could often be found pacing up and down the school corridors, meditating and reciting mumbled prayers, or singing his lines with his rosary in his hands. He was a good teacher and his Catholic orientation, together with his love of language, reminded me a lot of my own father. The two of them were actually old-time friends. Old Man Majola died a few years after I had left the school, and I was devastated when I heard. He was one of those gifted and special teachers who knew how to 'grow' a child into a student. Like so many others who passed through his hands, I feel blessed to have had him as one of my mentors, for he inspired me to take my passions of talking and writing seriously. He made me feel I had a gift for such things and through the close attention he paid to my words, helped me to understand better the mysteries of my own expression, and work for more meaning and depth in it.

In 1989, at the age of seventeen, I began my undergraduate degree in Social Sciences at the University of Natal in Durban. My majors were English, Sociology and Zulu, and I also took Linguistics and Psychology. At the time when I went to

University the floodgates of opportunity were opening for students from previously disadvantaged communities. It was a period when South Africa, with all its past divisions, was experiencing the initial phases of political and social transformation and the institutions were trying to reflect this reality. This was a time of heightened attack on political oppression, an era when the working-class was reorganising itself towards taking control over its life and rights. I went to University to learn about these changes, understand them and negotiate my way through them. I found the academic environment very stimulating and it was in this context that it became clearer to me what capitalism and racism were all about, and the deep scars that both had left on my society and country. I had always been attracted to issues of social change and community development. A Social Sciences qualification offered me the opportunity to study my society and better understand its dynamics, language and culture. My ambition was to play a meaningful role in the transformations and contribute towards making a real difference, particularly for 'my people' – the marginalised black population, whose lives had been badly disrupted by the years of political oppression.

I found campus life exciting and loved the experience of learning and interacting with a lot of other minds. After finishing my undergraduate degree in 1991, I proceeded to do my Honours in Sociology over the next two years. I felt I had to further my studies in order to expand my world view still more and apply what I had learnt in the outside world. I wanted to 'go' and 'grow', and discover new realities that could only add to my knowledge base. I was particularly thrilled by the experience of writing my Honours Dissertation, which explored the impact of non-governmental or community-based organisations on the development and survival of socially-impoverished communities in southern Africa. I did my research work in Maputaland, an underdeveloped rural area in northern KwaZulu-Natal. I enjoyed the fieldwork since it gave me the opportunity to test out the ideas and theories of development that I had been taught at University against the realities and practices of a 'real' developing society. The issue I was dealing with was one very close to my heart and I learnt an enormous amount in the process. I was thrilled to receive a good mark for the dissertation and graduated with pride.

In tandem with my studies, I was also employed by the University as a tutor and junior lecturer in Social Studies. Part of my task was to champion the establishment of a community infrastructure that would assist with identifying black students who had passed their matric exams, but who did not have enough points to gain automatic entry into University. This educational development programme was called Teach-Test-Teach (TTT). I managed a group of young extension officers and together we covered many kilometres, selecting and counselling potential students identified in the field. They were then taken through a rigorous full year's educational development programme that equipped them with the skills they needed to cope with tertiary study. I lectured in Sociology, Politics and Anthropology, while my colleagues handled the other courses. It was my choice to be part of the actual tutoring process, rather than simply delegating to others, since this allowed me to stand up and talk to a captive audience – I loved those lecturing and tutoring moments! TTT and the road soon became my second home, and I look back to those days with fondness.

The Teach-Test-Teach project was part of the University of Natal's Affirmative Action and Equity Strategy. TTT was a Distance Education Model, which meant that candidates had to learn on their own from their home bases and come in regularly to the University for tutorials and academic guidance. It was during this programme that I first noticed the true commitment of a black child from a disadvantaged background to his or her personal progress. Most of these students were from working-class families and underdeveloped community backgrounds, with very little money to spare for buying textbooks and paying for transport. Despite all these disabling factors, they were undeterred, determined to follow their dreams of success and escape the entrapping obstacles of their impoverished backgrounds. They came in their droves to the TTT office, walking on foot up the long hill to the University from where the buses dropped them at the bottom. Their enthusiasm was very exciting to me and made me want to work even harder to meet them halfway. They also formed self-directed study groups and met on their own initiative to study together and assist each other, often far away in small community halls, by the light of flickering candles and dim paraffin lanterns. Those who passed the TTT Entrance Exam, which was written at the end of the year, were accepted into University for study. But their mentoring continued, and I would meet some of them again in the Knowledge Development Foundation Course, which was designed to assist them with developing appropriate skills for survival in their chosen fields. Most of the candidates were very passionate about issues that related to the problems that faced developing communities in their own hometowns. It was not surprising to me that many chose a Social Sciences degree, since their interests lay in understanding social development and applying its theories and strategies towards upliftment in their own societies. These were very heady days for me. I loved my role as a junior lecturer and never missed a class. I was at the cutting edge of my youthful energies, only twenty years old and already rubbing shoulders with lecturers and tutors, deans and professors. I had developed a taste for status and power, and I was thoroughly enjoying the dance under the spotlight. Life was a cool cruise in the fast lane, and I was constantly on the run.

Towards the end of 1994, I left the University to join a mushroom-growing farm at Shongweni, a small rural settlement about 35 kms north of Durban. Tongaat Mushrooms, as the farm was called, was where the popular Denny Mushrooms were planted, grown, packed and sent to the market. I loved the serenity of the country environment around the farm and from the very first day, when I came for the interview, I knew that I wanted to 'grow my life' in that place. When the panel asked me why I felt I was the best candidate for the post, given that there were others with better qualifications and industrial relations experience who had also applied, my answer was: 'It is those who dare to take the first step and aspire to flight who one day *will* fly.' My confidence won me the job and in September 1994, I proudly took up my first corporate employment as the Personnel Officer at Tongaat Mushrooms.

My University studies had not only taught me about social relations, but also about the dynamics of industrial relations. Now I was getting the chance to put the theory into practice. I had enjoyed my University days, but the time had come to explore new fields and opportunities. In order to continue growing, I needed a job that could match my expanding ambitions. My new job description encompassed a broad range of functions, including the employment of staff, human resources development, handling of negotiations and industrial disputes, and ensuring that there were effective and open lines of communication between management and staff on the farm floor. There I was, working on a farm – a place of utmost worker subordination – fresh from a University job – a place of utmost intellectual freedom. It was an exciting contrast, but one which also left me a bit out of my depth. At first, I was concerned that I had not been trained to handle these functions, but I calmed myself with the memories of my TTT team and our experiences with the students – a process which in many ways had been a human resources exercise. In due time, I regained my balance and self-confidence and made friends with the other employees. I met the challenges one at a time, learning and perfecting my skills with each step I took.

I enjoyed my job at Mushrooms and found a lot of reward in the performance of my duties. This was a farm where not much had happened thus far to improve labour relations and upgrade worker skills. There was little to motivate worker effort and management constantly lamented the poor productivity. I helped to initiate some radical changes in the working conditions of the labour force and was happy that much was achieved in a short space of time. Part of what had facilitated the racial oppression in South Africa was the widespread practice whereby employers simply did not bother to specify or define the job descriptions and responsibilities of black employees – a deliberate strategy that enabled the exploitation of workers at less pay than they deserved and which also made it difficult to organise industrial action. The same was also true of the conditions at Mushrooms. To address this state of affairs was top of my priority list, and within three months, I had finished drafting the job descriptions of the entire workforce – an exercise that saw many workers receiving improved salaries as a result of a well-defined Job Grading System. The exercise was invaluable in other ways too, in that it forced each worker to define his or her own placement and role in the company within the parameters of what was expected of them, and also to interrogate for themselves what the company meant to them. This had amazing spin-offs for industrial relations in general. It brought people to an understanding that their work was not just for pay, but for self and community betterment. It also resulted in management becoming more involved in community needs.

Together with Nelson Dawede, the former Personnel Relations Officer, who was transferred to another section on my appointment, I also initiated training courses to improve technical skills and literacy levels. Many employees who had years of experience but no proof of competency were now issued with certificates that reflected their abilities and qualifications. All of this, I believed, would go a long way towards improving worker understanding and appreciation of their duties, as well as bettering their working conditions and supporting their demands for better pay in wage negotiations. I found it a very gratifying experience to have contributed to the development and enrichment of others.

Dawede became a good friend and he taught me a lot during my time at Mushrooms, including how to handle the older people at work. I had the educational qualifications, but Dawede, who had not studied beyond matric, had the experience – and in a sense, he 'grew' me. The adults here were of a different mindset from the students that I was used to dealing with, but Dawede reminded me that despite this difference, they shared one common feature with the students – they too needed someone to understand the limiting backgrounds they came from, and how this impacted on their drive for self-betterment and development. I worked very hard to fulfil the challenges I was confronted with and put my energies into bringing to life the initiatives that emerged out of the job description exercise. I always appreciated the fact that management was so amenable to the changes that Dawede and I introduced, welcoming our attempts to try new methods of improving relations and productivity.

Another item on my priority list was the lack of effective and open communication on the farm. I started working on a company newsletter that reflected the various components of the farm – from work to recreation, social issues and policy changes – and this became my pet project. I enjoyed writing about life around me and still remember those cold lonely nights of typing away – as well as the long, enjoyable evenings spent at Dawede's house in the suburbs of Hillcrest, chatting away. I miss those times and I miss my friend.

The initially tense industrial relations mood that prevailed when I joined Mushrooms had started to normalise. In the beginning, there were always strikes and confrontations – placards, insults, lockouts, agitation by shop stewards and union representatives. These were of a different tenor to the University strikes I was used to, that erupted now and again on the campus, characterised by explosive jeers, rude toyi-toyi lyrics and daring acts of youthfulness. This was proper warfare, the mass action of angry and very serious adults. I was young and out of my depth and didn't really know how to handle these situations. As Personnel Officer in a highly conflicted environment, I was put in the position of mediator, expected to bridge the divides and thrown very much in the deep end. When the workers went on strike, it was my task to sound out their grievances, defuse the issues and get them back to work again. As young and inexperienced as I was, it was not easy to face a farmful of angry adults in a mediator's role. Although I had the respect of the workers, who appreciated my youth and my commitment to my job, they were tough in confrontation, and it was hard at times to keep myself afloat in the waves of unrest. I learnt very quickly what approach was needed in such situations, and my advice to anyone who ever finds themselves in similar shoes is to leave the diplomacy bullshit at the door. Above all, don't patronise, and listen rather than talk; hear with respect what the workforce has to say – you can always give your side later. I grew up fast in the course of these events and learnt to handle these situations more skilfully and wisely. I spent a lot of time with the workforce, doing what they were doing, the better to understand the conditions in which they worked. With time, the tense mood eased and this sparked dialogue and a greater sense of trust. During my time at Mushrooms, Dawede and I made significant inroads in promoting communication between management and the labour force – but in the end, cat and dog will always have their differences. In a capitalist enterprise, a certain amount of conflict is inevitable, and one has to realise and accept this. Nonetheless, it felt good to be involved in processes that assisted with changing people's lives, impressing on them that a change in conditions is only possible if we come together in genuine goodwill and tap into each others' psyches and potentials. It was my determined desire to make Mushrooms a model of good labour relations, to unlock the full potential of the farm and create an environment conducive to both productivity and friendly interactions. I had only been in my position for close on ten months, but I was on a roll – 'Director of Human Resources' was my dream, and already it seemed almost within my grasp.

Everything was going incredibly well for me. I had a good job, a significant salary, and I was the proud owner of my first car, a light blue 1.8 CTI Golf Sport. Only four months after I joined the farm as a Personnel Officer, I received a notch in position, and my office door boasted a shiny new sign that said 'Senior Personnel Manager'. My personal life was also going well and I was in the process of sharing wedding dreams with my girlfriend of two and a half years. A week before the crash, my employer informed me that I was earmarked for a promotion, which would entail a move to Head Office in Johannesburg – the Place of Gold. Ever since I was a child, I had dreamed of living my life in a place where the streets are 'paved with gold' and mansions await those who believe in themselves and in their potential to move the world. To me, Johannesburg was this very place, and I could already see myself reaching out to unlock the doors that lead to her chambers of prosperity and fulfilment. My self-confidence was at an all-time high. I was just 23, and already 'the world was my oyster', as they say. My dreams were in the process of transforming themselves into reality, new opportunities were opening up to me as fast as I could seize them and the sky was the limit. I had worked very hard to get where I was and I felt I deserved my success. Then suddenly ... like a broken promise, my life was turned upside down. All the glittering doors slammed shut, and my dreams lay dashed to pieces at my feet ...

## *Running Away*

I am running away
From this world of lost moments
From these tears I forever cry
And these tomorrows of my sorrows
Change has painted my skies in grey
And stolen the silver lining from my cloud

I am running away from it all
These questions inside my mind
This heavy doubt that hangs over my head
Where is the man I used to be?
And the boy that could jump over mountains?
What about the dream to express the dreams inside?

The hero and the warrior are in pain
I'm running away . . .

I am lighting candles in the wind
Hoping for a moment that is never going to be
For the hands of time to reverse away the past
And give back to me what has been stolen
How can life give to me only the pain?
The winds of change have blown away my house

I am running away
The knight and his armour are lost in the plain

I am running away from the pain
From my broken heart that bleeds
How will I face the future in my darkness?
Somebody help me I just can't take this
These walls that have imprisoned my soul
There is a storm brewing on the horizon

Change has painted my skies in grey
Where is the man I used to be?
Where is my knight and my warrior on these plains?
How can life give to me only the pain?
All I see is a storm that brews on the horizon

The hero and the warrior are slain
I'm running away . . .

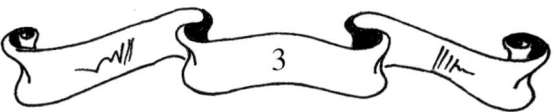

# 3

Paralysis . . . I was paralysed! It was a devastating realisation. It is hard to describe the feelings that went through me, the depth of my despair, how lost and alone I felt. I did not want to believe that such a thing had happened to me. Young as I was, I had already accomplished so much in my life and was looking forward to achieving so much more. I was at the peak of my potential, in the process of spreading my wings for still greater heights. My goal was to vault into the skies and shine up there with all the other stars. It was a crushing blow to realise that those big ambitions had died in the wreck along with the person I used to be. 'What about my dreams – is this where the road ends for me?' was all I could think of. I only had questions, but no solutions, nor any sense of direction to guide me out of my present crisis. I suppose I was just reeling from the blow, drowning in the pool of my own fears. It's not every day that you are faced with change on such a scale and it's hard to maintain equilibrium and an optimistic outlook under such circumstances. I used to cry a lot during those early days – most of the time alone, so as to hide my pain from others. It was all so strange and confusing.

I could not feel my lower body at all. My legs were numb and cold as ice. I had no control over my bladder and bowels. I was on a permanent catheter and had to wear a nappy – I was torn apart by the indignity of my condition and the helplessness I felt. There was a button next to my bed that I had to press to summon a staff member when I had messed myself, and every time it happened, I just could not bring myself to make the move. Finally, I would find the courage and with quaking hands press for help. Every time the nurses came to change my nappy and bedding, I would lie there frozen and wish for the moment to pass quickly. The nurses were always kind, but I couldn't deal with the fact that my privacy was suddenly invaded and my pride shattered. I would lie in my shame and wonder if that's the way a child feels every time he or she messes up – except that I was 23 years old! Every minute of every day I was confronted by some new and traumatic revelation. I was devastated to learn that I had also lost my erection in the accident. Short of a miracle, it was another loss I was going to have to live with for the rest of my life, and the pain of that realisation was not easy to take.

Early morning bed-baths, physiotherapists, occupational therapists, psychologists, neurologists, medical specialists and their assistants; white walls and ever-clean lab coats, tilt-tables and parallel bars, catheters and suppositories, X-rays and thermometers, multiple scans and timed visits . . . persistent wails and death in the ward. These were the elements that made up my days – not my version of an ideal world! Nobody wants to live in a place where death and life are continually balanced on the scales, and that has been my experience of what defines a hospital. In that place, there was constant pain and uncertainty, and the only thing that ever seemed to make any of the patients smile from the heart was the moment when they were discharged. I am scared of hospitals. I hate the way that control is taken away from you there. In that world, not much seems to be perceived as a positive sign. You wake up sad one morning and they say you are depressed; you wake up feeling more cheerful the following day and somebody says you are exhibiting signs of schizophrenia – you can almost hear their minds whispering 'denial'. You are constantly labelled and tagged. I hated living as a 'case': 'Sister, how is "he" today?' You become a third person in your very presence. 'Tell him such and such and make sure he takes this medication once in the morning and once before he sleeps.' My life was suddenly placed in someone else's hands in the name of care, my independence taken away from me. I felt I had lost myself. I was half out of my mind with fury at my situation, carried through the days on the waves of my frustration.

    I have never been one for confines – the outside world is my home, my space. Now, day after day, I was in bed, inside a ward with virtually no colour, no visual stimulation, where almost everything was white, from the ceiling above my head to the tiles on the floor below the white bed – all much too clean and antiseptic for an outdoors boy like me. All I wanted was to walk out that door back to my familiar 'pig-sty' at home. Even the food was very different from what I was used to in taste and appearance. The mood and the air was always cold. I take my hat off to the healthcare workers of the world for the hard work they put into trying to make those places a normal environment, where people can embrace the hope that they will live to see the next day in. Not that I was even in a bad hospital. Since I was fortunate enough to be on medical aid when the accident happened, the ambulance crew took me straight to a private health facility. This was Entabeni, a private hospital of world-class standard, where everything possible is done to ensure the highest levels of health and recovery. All the facilities were there to give a solid foundation to the long-term rehabilitation programme that would be implemented in the days ahead.

    I remember my reaction when the wheelchair first came – I cried my soul out. 'God, why have you forsaken me?' Questions and endless tears! The nursing staff helped me up and placed me on this 'object'. I hated it with all my heart – to me it represented my helplessness. My pride made it difficult for me to accept. I could not deal with the prospect of being seen riding on that thing by people who had known me during my able-bodied days. I kept being told everything would be 'fine' – but to me, that wheelchair tolled the bells of my final moment. I was so traumatised by the thought of lifelong paralysis that I believed I was literally going to die. At night, I had recurring bad dreams where I was drowning in the bathtub. My legs were paralysed and my arms too weak to pull me up and save me from the danger – I would actually see myself slipping away underwater. It was a terrible nightmare. When I woke up there would be beads of sweat running down my forehead. I know now that the dream represented the helplessness I was feeling, but at the time, it all seemed terribly real. I would lie there dead scared – convinced it could really happen and that it would be the end of me. I longed to go home where I knew I would be safe with the people that loved me. I was very lonely in that hospital ward, a stranger in a strange world – isolated from my own identity and the vital energy of society. I admit I wasn't an ideal patient. I threw a few tantrums and boycotted meals in protest. It was the only way I could express my frustration at the situation in which I found myself. In a short space of time, my temper had created bad blood between me and some of the nursing staff.

One of the most devastating things about paralysis is the way it impacts on normal bodily functions. Because I could no longer urinate in the normal way, I had to use a catheter to empty my bladder. The first few days, I was hooked up to a permanent tube. Then I graduated to the disposable kind, which I was supposed to insert myself. I hated that bloody catheter. It became my worst enemy. I found it completely humiliating to have to fiddle with myself, poking about in my penis, trying to insert the tube into the right channel. It was like puncturing the very essence of your manhood, tampering with the core of you. I made up my mind to boycott it, convinced there had to be another way. With my very limited understanding of human anatomy, it seemed to me that if water could pass into my bladder unaided, it must eventually, by the sheer pressure of its own gravity, expel itself unaided. I decided to conduct a little experiment to prove my theory. After two days of not urinating, my bladder swelled up till I looked like someone in the early stages of pregnancy. My doctor wasn't happy with what I was doing, warning me that I was creating a serious risk of infection, with all the complications this would bring. But I stubbornly persevered. On the third day, I woke up to find the bed soaking wet and my bladder blissfully empty. I lay there laughing in joy. My small triumph over the catheter signalled a much bigger victory in other ways. The lesson it taught me was to work with and listen to my body. After three months of battling through this messy procedure of allowing my bladder to fill naturally and then pressurise itself to empty naturally, I began to get control over the process. I started to feel the subtle pulsating that warned me my bladder needed to empty itself. Through this experience, my mind learnt to attune itself to other signals too, the slight spasms in the legs, the tingling sensations in the feet that indicated that all was not as it should be. In this way, I developed a much more harmonious relationship with my body in general, and my capacity for sensation has come back to an amazing degree.

One of the things I found so difficult about being bedridden was that aside from the paralysis and a few minor injuries sustained in the accident, I was in good health. My body was incapacitated, but free from pain and full of vitality, and my mind was still operating with all its former drive and energy. One of the big frustrations eating at me was the belief that I was doomed to a wheelchair's pace of locomotion forever. When I first learnt I was paralysed, I was terrified by the thought that my driving days were over. My family showed me photographs of my beloved Golf, which I had been driving at the time of the crash. I was horrified by the wreckage I saw and completely devastated by the thought that it had been my first and last car. I had loved that Golf like a part of me. I bought it on the 30th of August 1994 and the very next day it emerged from a Car Audio Shop, equipped with an uncompromising sound system. Off we went together – a marriage made in boys' heaven. I cared for that car with absolute dedication, kept it polished, vacuumed and serviced – in mint condition. The two of us had a wonderful relationship that was tragically terminated after only nine months by the collision with the fateful brick wall. We both suffered the heavy blows of impact and my baby was towed away to a scrapyard while I was being wheeled into the ICU – two lives forever separated.

As the days of bed-ridden immobility rolled by, all I wanted to do was get up, walk back into my life, find myself another car and drive away to my dreams. I was terribly frustrated by the thought that my crucial independence had been permanently revoked. This was why I hated the wheelchair so much – it could never substitute for the class of wheels I loved. When a gorgeous occupational therapist visited me at Entabeni Hospital one day the first question I posed to her was: 'Will I ever be able to drive a car again?' When she said 'yes' with a bright smile and explained how it was possible, relief gushed through me. I had never seen anyone in a wheelchair driving a car and up to that point had no idea that it was even a viable option. I came to see for myself just how possible it was when, a short while later, I met Vusi Ndimeni, a compassionate stranger who took an interest in me and was later to become my good friend and brother. Our meeting was one of those fortunate co-incidences that life throws across your path. It was a few months after the crash, and I was experiencing severe pains down my back. Since I had already left the hospital, a friend recommended I see a chiropractor, so I made an appointment and got someone to take me along. Wheeling myself into the consultation room, I noticed an African guy sitting on a sofa. We did not even greet each other, and when I came out he was gone. A lady at the reception desk informed me that 'the stranger' had asked for my number so he could phone me later. I asked why he wanted to contact me, but all she said was, 'He just wants to talk to you.' Later that evening 'a Vusi' called and told me that he was also in a wheelchair. He remarked that he could not help but notice the sorrow that was registered all over my face. Strangely enough, it did not even occur to me to tell him to go to hell, which was my favourite response at that time to anyone in a wheelchair who tried to come close to me. Instead, I opened up and told Vusi that I was not fine. I confided to this stranger that my life was a mess and that the changes I was faced with had completely demolished me. All of this I said with tears streaming down my face. Vusi's response was: 'All will be fine with time.' It was the same response I'd heard over and over again from others and it usually sent me into a rage. But in Vusi's mouth, it sounded different. He had really listened to my pain. He knew what it was to be in the place I was in, and when he told me everything would be all right, I believed him.

Vusi's paralysis was the result of a bullet hitting his spine in an incident related to his work with prisoners. He was strong, positive and reassuring. He told me that it only needed positive thinking for me to make it through this disaster. The sincerity in his voice was very convincing and there was something about him that I could not ignore. I felt very comfortable talking with him and found security in knowing that there was someone out there who had felt and understood my pain. He invited me to his home to meet his wife and child. The following day, my brothers took me to his house in the grounds of Westville Prison, where he worked as a prison warder. It was during that visit that things fell into place for me. Vusi was driving a maroon BMW 325I, complete with sports kit and a low suspension that exaggerated its sleek, sporty lines – a real beauty specially designed to meet his needs. He took me for a drive and later allowed me to try the mounted hand controls. When I drove that car, it was like heaven had opened its doors for me to come in and rest in peace. I knew then that it was completely possible for me to drive, despite my paralysis, and the new dream I started to embrace right then and there was to get my own wheels and drive myself wherever I wanted to go.

After a full month of being confined to my hospital bed, I had my first chance to venture into the outside world. I was given a weekend pass-out, which allowed me to spend the weekend at home and return to the hospital on Monday morning. The date was the 20th of May – I remember it well because it was the same day that I heard on the news that actor Christopher Reeves, the Superman hero, had broken his neck in a horse-riding accident. My friend Bonga Mlambo collected me, driving a car identical to the Golf in which I had crashed. It was a freaky co-incidence and it unsettled me terribly. I clearly remember the fear I felt of being in that car, made worse by my lack of physical control. I had minimal balance at that time, very little command over my posture. As we drove away from the hospital, the first place I asked to be taken to was the infamous 'wall' – the crash site in Umbilo Road. It was a strange feeling of *déjà vu* to be recreating the fateful journey in the identical car. I still had absolutely no memory of what had happened, yet in the space of a month, my whole life had turned upside down.

Arriving home was a very moving experience. My brothers (I include my close cousins in the term) were overjoyed to see me. We sat and chatted on the balcony like old times. But when darkness fell, they had to take me inside. My body thermostat had gone completely haywire. Even though the evening was warm, I was freezing, unable to warm up no matter how many blankets they piled on me. That visit home started me thinking deeply. So much had changed in the time of my absence; I no longer had the freedom of the house. I watched my brothers bounding up and down the stairs that lead to the outside room we had shared and felt for the first time the cruel contrast between their freedom of movement and my confinement. I was no longer master of my own fate. If I wanted something, someone had to fetch it for me. If I wanted to go to bed, somebody had to carry me there. It was during that weekend that it truly dawned on me that this was not a temporary state of affairs, but my permanent condition. I remember that I started to cry. The next day, the whole family came to see me; they gathered around me – my father, mother, sisters, and brothers – solicitous and loving, so eager to be of service, to fetch me this or do that for me. I was completely touched by their loving attention. I wasn't used to being the family focal point. They were behaving like the admiring audiences who used to gather round me during my Michael Jackson days to watch my dancing displays. In some ways, their loving attention made my new situation even harder to bear. But it was a good pain – a reminder to me that I wasn't alone, but part of a loving community.

   I slept well that night, happy to be home. In the morning, when I woke up, it was to find that I had messed myself. My brothers and my friend Tobias took it in their stride. As if it was the most natural thing in the world, they carried me through to the bathroom, cleaned me up and changed the bedding. Throughout that visit, I was overwhelmed by the extent of the love and acceptance my brotherhood showered on me. There was never any sense that they were doing things out of pity for my helpless state, or that I was a dependant they had to take care of. They related to me like a favourite celebrity, fussed around me with genuine solicitousness, competed with each other to push my wheelchair, and generally made me feel special. Again and again they proved to me that they were not just friends and brothers in name, but in soul.

   On the Saturday, at my request, I was driven to the scrapyard to pay my last respects to the wreckage of my car. The sight of it completely shocked me. My Golf had been transformed into a little Coke can. All the windows were shattered, the metal buckled and tangled, the steering column mangled, the driver's seat ripped to pieces. It seemed incredible that anyone could have remained alive in that wreck, and brought home to me the full miracle of my survival.

   Monday dawned, and with it, the terrible moment of having to return to the hospital. There were lots of tears all round. There and then I made a promise to my brothers that there would be no more pass-outs; the next time I left the hospital, it would be for good. The weekend at home had given me just the incentive I needed. I went back to the ward with new determination, started exercising and generally gearing myself towards getting off my bed. I had been told by the doctors that I would need to remain in hospital for eight months before I could start thinking about rehabilitation programmes. There was a lot of swelling around the spine in the region of the snapped T6 vertebra, which would need time to heal. I had other ideas, however. I wasn't prepared to keep lying there day after day watching my life waste away. I couldn't see the necessity. Now that my fractured collar bone and other minor injuries had healed, I had no pain. Aside from the paralysis I was in good health. I had no objection to visiting the hospital for my rehab sessions, but I couldn't see the necessity for remaining there for another seven months. As far as I was concerned, there were enough practitioners on the outside who could monitor my progress just as capably. One week after my pass-out, five weeks in total after my admission, I took the liberty of discharging myself. I think there were a few secret sighs of relief when I left; including from my neurologist. In my frustrations I had put him through a lot of uphill. He represented to me the pitiless face of what had happened to me, the implacable clinical voice of decision that pronounced the hard facts and commanded from a height. He was a top-class physician, but his bedside manner tended to be lacking in the human touch. He was not one for physical contact, preferring to instruct from a distance and leave it to others to carry out the ministrations at close quarters. His depersonalised style often infuriated me, for it made me feel like an object. There were many times that I tried to provoke him into losing his temper with me, so that I would have the excuse to unleash my bottled rage. But no matter what the provocation, he remained the gentleman, always sidestepping confrontation, refusing to rise to the bait. When I complained to him about the lack of privacy in the ward I was in, saying that I needed my space and demanding to be transferred elsewhere, he looked at me in his unsmiling way and simply said: 'But you told me you belonged to the people!' It is to his great credit that after all the churlish and childish behaviour I had thrown at him, he could still remain sincerely concerned for my well-being and say to me when I left: 'If anything happens, just remember that we're here for you.'

    I was in a very upbeat mood the day I left the hospital, laughing, shaking hands with the staff, cracking jokes. Many of them, I'm sure, were glad to see the back of me, but I think there was a degree of regret as well. The matron's comment to me was that if there had been such a thing as a hospital hall of fame, I would be in it. This was in reference to the huge numbers of visitors who constantly streamed in to see me during my time there, including two busloads of Tongaat Mushrooms employees. Their presence was important to me, made me feel like the world still cared. They transformed the bleak hospital ward into something vibrant and alive, that had the energy of a Rock Concert. The life and gaiety they brought into that cold space spilled over to the other patients. There were some grumbles at first, but my neighbour on the one side – a typical 'grumpy old white man' – summed up the general feeling when he said: 'It's good to have some life and laughter brightening up this dreary place. Let's just accept it and be happy.'

    On the 30th of May 1995, I wheeled myself out of the hospital doors into the bright sunshine of freedom. There was only one mission in my mind: to recover, whatever it took, get back in the driver's seat of my life again and regain the scattered wealth that I felt I had been robbed of. I still at that stage cherished the dream that I would one day walk again, and I took it for granted that I'd soon have my old job back. Senior management had paid me a visit in hospital, and I'd been very anxious to prove to them how fine I was. One of the first things I did after I got out was to go and pay a visit to my second home – Mushrooms. I asked my mother to take me, which she willingly agreed to do. It was an electrifying experience. As we drove in, I was spotted by one of the employees, who instantly dropped everything and ran to spread the word. The entire workforce turned out to greet me, pouring like ants from every corner of the farm to mob the car. They welcomed me back like a prodigal son, not just a colleague. One of the managers remarked that they'd had VIPs and politicians visiting before, but no one had ever brought the farm to a standstill like I did that day.

The esteem and love in which I was so obviously held made it all the more difficult to accept my termination. This was enacted two months after the crash, when senior management informed me that they would be retiring me on the basis of ill-health. There were a few considerations that had pushed them to reach this decision. The primary one was that they felt I would not be able to cope with my workload, given my condition. Secondly, they felt that my rehabilitation programme, which was quite intense, was going to clash with my job commitment. And last but not least, they felt that I was going to find it hard in a purely logistical sense to do my job, since the physical environment at Mushrooms, with its sectioned layout and many steps, was not conducive to wheelchair access. This would leave me virtually confined to my office and make it difficult for me to move about freely from section to section as my job required. I acknowledge that their concerns were not without foundation. But I felt that the decision was premature. At the very least, I wanted the chance to prove that I could cope and with time find my feet. Employment is a major rehabilitation factor to a disabled individual. I could only accept, however, that my employers felt differently and that their decision had been made in good faith, whether I agreed with it or not. The management at Mushrooms had always been good to me. They had taken me on as a raw recruit, had given me the chance to exercise my potential and had allowed me a lot of latitude. In the nine months that I'd worked there, I'd learnt an enormous amount and had developed both intellectually and as a person. I found it incredibly difficult to leave the farm, not just because of the employment, but because the place had become my second family, with everybody in it a valued part of my life. I cried when the decision was announced and was left feeling very torn apart by this turn of events.

Mushrooms did what they could to cushion the blow, ensuring that financially at least, I was well taken care of. They informed me that the company would pay me a pension until I died. It was small consolation to me at the time, however. The idea of early retirement was a terrible concept to me. I was only 23 years old, full of sap, as they say, and with my whole life still ahead of me. Before the crash, I had had a very bright future to look forward to, big dreams to reach towards and the determination and ability to make them happen. Those dreams were now suddenly snatched away from me, and all I was left holding onto was a pay slip at the end of every month that labelled me a pensioner. To me, pensioners were old people who sat at home complaining about everything and counting the crazy flies that crack their heads against the window panes in a bid to escape. I was horrified by the thought that I had been turned into one of them. I wanted to scream out loud – 'O Heart of Mine!' – like in the words of the Boz Scaggs song:

> You will never understand the reason why
> Heart of Mine
> How will you keep from dying
> Stop reminiscing . . .

I felt completely shattered in every way, unfairly punished by life for circumstances that were not of my making. Everything seemed to be slipping through my fingers, including my heart.

## *The House Is Lonely*

The house is lonely
and I am all by myself
The curtains are drawn
and no ray of light shines into my corner

The colour of the sky is grey
and on my windowpane I see raindrops
The storm is raging in the clouds
and I am the candle in the wind

My soul is empty
and only yesterday I had found you
We played in the water that sunny day
and at night we embraced and fell in love

The phone is quiet
and only one voice can lift me high
Tender words from lips so soft and thin
That turn and twist at a stolen touch of a kiss

The night is still
and all the stars are deep in sleep
Only an owl hoots its message of sadness
Loneliness can drive you to madness

The house is lonely
The colour of the sky is grey
My soul is empty
The phone is quiet
The night is still
– and I miss you . . .

# 4

She was the love of my life and only eighteen when we met – very beautiful; she completely took my breath away. When I said I loved her, it was straight from my heart. We were everything to each other, friends as well as lovers; her secrets were mine and mine were known only to her. We taught each other a lot, travelled places together ... shared everything. I still recall our first kiss, her 'sweet lips soft as petals'; it was the 21st of June 1993. It is no exaggeration to say that for me, she was the sky and all the stars in it, daytime and the night. When the accident happened, even though it changed everything for us, I just could not find it in me to say goodbye and let her go.

After I lost my job at Mushrooms, my love life started taking a crash-bound path. I felt out of control with everything and feared the worst if she exited my life. It was difficult for her, because I was no longer the man I used to be; it was not just my ability to walk that was lost, but a lot of others things. Disability steals away your sexual performance, and with that, your sense of confidence and control. I remember lying in hospital and asking her to leave me and find another; but she said no and cried heart-rending tears. I held her in my arms and promised her that I would try my best to beat the odds and bounce back, that it would be like old times again; she held onto me tightly. Looking back now, I think it was not very kind of me to ask her to leave me. But I had to. I knew that my disability was going to be a tough path for a young girl to walk. It was not my wish to see her suffer – I loved her and knew she loved me too. I also remember the first night we spent together after I had left the hospital – she said she wanted to be with me. I could not get an erection and when I attempted masturbation to stimulate my penis, it only triggered my bladder and I wet the bed. My God – how it blew me apart! I could have killed myself right then and there. I was totally embarrassed and could not even look her in the eyes – I just cried. But she was a strong woman, despite her youth, and she took the disaster lightly. She cleaned me up and assured me that things would be okay with time; but I knew in my heart that I was slowly losing the battle.

As my dreams of holding onto this woman began to fade, I became more possessive of her, agitated and suspicious. I would constantly wonder where she was and with whom. I would torture myself with thoughts such as: 'I wonder who she's kissing now?' Our relationship took a lot of strain and in the end it fell apart. I was quick to shift the blame – I felt let down by her. The truth is that the situation was hard for her in its own right, and I was not making it any easier. At that stage, my behaviour made it almost impossible for her and others to live with me. I was preoccupied with my walking days and my sexuality, and forgot that there is more to me and to love than my ability to walk, my penis and my performance in bed. When the affair finally crashed, I crashed with it. Sorrow engulfed me and I cried all the tears I had. Despair became the dark veil through which I viewed life. 'How Can You Mend A Broken Heart?' I would ask, in the words of the Teddy Pendergrass song, 'All I need is to find somebody to hold me! Please help me mend my broken heart!' In my fantasy, I would reach out my arms, hoping for some good Samaritan to come along and change the situation that had me trapped and pinned against the walls of my own self-pity. I wrote poems in which I described my lonely nights as 'a haunted town of lost dreams, where distant owls hoot a message of sadness'.

The only way to ease the lonely pain I felt was to sedate myself with the soothing music of songs. I used to sing endlessly about finding love, wonderful love. My dreams were about experiencing that gentle touch once more, the touch of love. I had found it and lost it. Listening to music gave me hope and opened my heart, healing the scars and bruises. With time I healed and accepted the pain . . .

I needed to revisit the world and mix with people again. But the thought of leaving the house was very frightening to me. I still find it difficult to explain those feelings – the emotions of fear, anger, sadness and hopelessness that held me captive. At times, I would give vent to them in explosive tantrums, spilling out my frustrations on anyone in range. I felt completely let down by life and I was taking it all out on those who least deserved it, the people I was closest to. I became unreasonably jealous of others, and often wished in my bitterness that the calamity had happened to them and not to me. There were days when I hated everybody and wanted only to be left to myself. A lot of my bitterness was directed at myself. I was tortured by the difference in image between what I used to be and what I had become. I hated the wheelchair, the catheters and those bloody nappies. I hated everyone who asked me how I was and felt like breaking into tiny pieces every time anybody said to me that 'things are going to be fine'. I was on fire with helpless rage, burning away, and it seemed to me that no one else could feel the heat.

The thought of being associated with disability was a ghost that haunted my every waking minute. There was a nagging sense of shame, as if I had committed some inexcusable offence, as if it was somehow my fault that I had allowed myself to be dumped into a zone that nobody wanted to be associated with. I had grown up in a society loaded with negative stereotypes and misconceptions about disability. I remembered the days at school, when disabled students were never an integral part of the environment. They never participated in sport or anything else and did not have many friends. I recalled how, on my many walks through the city, the only time I ever encountered disabled figures was when I saw them at the street corners – begging. I hated being a part of this category of people and I loathed my disability. I had always belonged to the mainstream, and now I felt shunted onto the sidewalk; it was simply too heavy a burden for a boy of 23 to bear. For a time, I turned to the bottle to drown my sorrows. I binged myself to laughter, and in that way, escaped myself for a while . . .

In the beginning, I still had hope that I would walk again. In my dreams, I was always walking, jumping or dancing energetically, or running around. The mornings after these dreams were always terrible because reality would sink in and the contrast would be too painful to bear. All I wanted was to be the person I used to be, the person I could only now be in my dreams. It was not easy to wake up to find the sheets and mattress wet, my nappy soiled and my legs twitching in spasms. The thought that all this had happened and I could not feel it or control it, killed me more. I wanted nothing to do with any of it. I suppose this was the reason why I did not want to meet with other people living with disabilities. I remember when a representative from Disabled People of South Africa phoned to say he would like to pay me a visit. I told him in no uncertain terms to forget it and demanded that he respected my privacy. The silence that followed over the phone told me that we understood each other only too well. I was very harsh with him and did not even thank him or bid him a respectful goodbye. He never phoned again. I regret my behaviour now, but at that time I simply did not want to be a part of the disabled experience; medical people and psychologists term a reaction such as mine 'denial'. It was only in time that it slowly dawned on me that my state of affairs was permanent and my walking days were only still alive in my dreams.

It became increasingly clear that I couldn't continue to hide myself away forever. In order to resume my life, I had to leave the protection of the house and face the changing weathers of outside society. But my fear of being out in public places made me very insecure about leaving home. The first few months after I left the hospital, I remained inside the house, only venturing out after dark. When I was out, I always made sure that my brothers were hanging around me. I felt extremely uneasy if they were even a few yards away – let alone out of sight. I would imagine people were looking at me and noticing disasters that I wasn't yet aware of. But whether it was true that they were looking at me, or whether it was just my mind fearing that something might happen to embarrass me in full view of the public, I can't say. I still had spasms down my legs and limited control over my bowels and bladder, and this made me feel very insecure. I remember that about two weeks after I came out of hospital, friends threw me a party; I made a brief appearance and without warning, made a speedy exit. I felt so uncomfortable and so alone in the company of all those hundreds of people. Life was a rollercoaster in those days. There were times when everything seemed fine, and I took refuge in the love I received from those around me. Then there were other times, long days when nothing mattered and I would pull back into my small corner of sorrows and darkness. I would not ever wish to live through those times again; they were the most difficult episodes of my life. However, I believe that those setbacks and mind-shattering moments were what taught me to be open and accepting of pain. I felt sorry for myself and sometimes cried uncontrollably. And yet, even in the worst moments, something in me was determined not to give up.

After almost half a year of pain and trauma and continual wishing for a miracle, I realised that my family and close friends were beginning to lose hope that they would ever see me flash my smiles again. My sorrow was affecting their lives as well as mine. It was especially hard on my father, an internationally respected social scientist, who had taken great pride in watching his first-born son following in his footsteps. He was almost completely shattered by the accident and went an extra thousand miles to meet every one of my needs. He left me in no doubt of his love for me. Every Wednesday, he accompanied me to my physiotherapy sessions, where I attempted steps with the aid of parallel bars and took a dive in a heated pool. I suppose he just wanted to see his boy walking and active again; he so much wanted to see me happy. But the pressure of his hopes sometimes made it more difficult. I knew he meant well, but his interference sometimes drove me to distraction. 'Have you done your exercises?' he would ask me, at a time when I was exercising myself half to death in my determination to get mobile again. He would nag me to take my tablets, as if I couldn't decide to do it for myself, or chide me about coming home late, not understanding how much I needed to be out there in the world, that my soul's survival depended on it. Inevitably, his interference led to fights between us. I know now that I was wrong to construe his actions as possessive and over-protective, when he only meant to be understanding and loving. But I was in pieces at the time, able to see nothing but my own pain, disintegrating in the whirlwinds of change.

My whole family was very cut up by the accident and wanted to see me happy again. My mother was very strong; I suppose one does not become a nurse in a hospital if one does not have the guts to box with tragedy. My mother is someone who believes that healing comes with a positive mind and she will push anyone towards realising that philosophy. She nursed me with gentleness but blew her top at times when she thought I was dragging along aimlessly. I knew she was hurting for me, but unlike my old man, she did not show it so openly. My mother and I have always been very close and my disability drew us even closer. My little sisters did their utmost to cheer me up – Nana and Khethiwe cooking my meals, with Thulisile constantly asking if there was anything I needed. They frequently came to my room to challenge me to games of Scrabble in the hope of taking my mind off its troubles. They also did their fair share of 'counselling' – and for that I will always be grateful to 'my little angels'.

My big twin sisters were also there for me and always encouraged me to look on the positive side of things and hope for a brighter tomorrow. I was lucky that most of my questions – medical and general – could be met with informative answers. This is because one of the twins, Babongile, is a medical doctor and she advised me that I should never bottle things up but always feel free to speak my mind to her. She gave me all the time I needed and also allowed me to cry. In her, I had someone I could really talk to, someone I could trust with my secrets and fears. Her twin sister, Bongiwe, who had married four months before the crash and moved to Cape Town, came home regularly to check up on me. It was always a pleasure when she appeared. Bongiwe and I were big buddies when we were growing up, listening to Heavy Metal together and walking long distances through the suburbs to buy LPs from the shopping mall a few kilometres from the University. She asked me to speak on behalf of her siblings and to present her culturally to her 'new family' at her wedding, a duty that I felt honoured to perform. A few months after the crash, she and her husband presented me with a nephew, and that event gave me a wonderful chance to watch life blossoming through all its stages of growth, from embryo to fully-formed human being. The event gave me a new perspective and made me see that just like a baby that grows and develops in its own time, so I too was learning the ways of my new life. That child was a blessing to me in many ways, for as he crawled about and balanced on everything and anything to reach his targets and find what he wanted, I also learnt to do the same. I started crawling out of bed to fetch this and that – balancing on chairs to lift myself up and reach table tops – and crawling back again. That small baby gave me a reason to reach out, stretch myself and progress.

My brothers embraced me with the full warmth of their support and made it their personal mission to see to my happiness and recovery. 'Don't fall too far down/You are not the only one/Don't let it hurt so bad' was Luther Vandross's advice in a ballad that my younger brother Thabani played for me on the jukebox. What a direct message! I felt those lines with every fibre of my being. One of my great fears when the tragedy struck was that I was no longer going to be the big brother role model to my army of siblings. I so badly wanted to be someone that my brothers could look up to. I needn't have worried, however. For as I rose and fell through the phases of my changes, their respect for me grew stronger. It was their encouragement that enabled me to deal with my new realities in a truthful, constructive and positive way. This was what my young brother was reminding me of with the song he played for me. The boys also assisted with my physical exercises and ensured that I was included in everything, so that I never felt that my condition had taken away any opportunities or possibilities from me. It was my brothers who lifted me when I was down and almost out: 'He ain't heavy, he's my brother' – that is a song I will always love because it rings so true for me, reminding me of my love for my own brothers.

During those dark and isolated days, there was never a time when a friend from the good old days was not around. These were the people with whom I had shared some of the most memorable moments of my life – people that I had known from a long time back, coming to me to reassure me that they still stood by me and that 'it would all be all right'. 'Friends will be friends' the Queen song says, and these friends more than lived up to the trust I put in them. Theirs were the listening ears that had received some of my most intimate questions, the willing mouths that were always ready to pour out advice and tribute to me; the accepting silence that knew my deep secrets; the light that always saw me through the storms. All of them had the same thing to say to me: 'Believe, and everything will fall into place.' I was such a pain at that time, and my outbursts were all too often directed at them. But still they kept coming, from distances both close and far away, showing the true mettle of friendship. Their loyalty posed a particular challenge to me; it put me under obligation not to disappoint the faith they had in me. I had to do something to repay all of them for their unwavering support, prayers and hopes. So I dumped the whisky and smashed the brandy bottle – pulled myself up out of my spiral of self-pity and vowed to my friends never to bow down to failure again.

But the love of friends and family, however supportive they are, isn't enough. In order to recover my self-respect, I had to engage the world again. And that meant taking the first step and putting myself out there for others to find me. As the cycle of time drifted on and happiness cautiously circled back, I found myself wanting to win back my sense of independence and control. I had always been a very visible young man and I needed to taste that social recognition again. In September '95 – five months after the crash – I bought myself a bright red BMW 3.25is Evolution 2 – a model that is particularly revered by the township boys. Their name for the car is *'iGusheshe'* – a word that is hard to translate but which evokes the aura of God himself. A bolder statement than that red *iGusheshe* it was not possible to make! When I sat inside this car for the first time and drove it away, I felt a tingling sense of fulfilment throughout my being. I had achieved a longheld dream and this boosted my confidence dramatically. But the significance of the car went even deeper. The message of that moment was that disability had not stolen everything away from me. I had always been a fast mover – in all senses of the term – delighting in speed, in a race, in outdoing the competition. The *iGusheshe*, with its sports car design, offered me just that – a symbolic race against the lost life, a race against time to recover my advantage, my winning edge, while it was still possible. I was feeling strong, revved up to go again, red with ambition. This car was the physical embodiment of my emotional state of mind, reflecting my own metaphoric evolution from chairbound immobility to 'airborn' flight. In many ways, I had not yet overcome the anger and loss inside me. I was moving through a phase, searching for my identity – crashing and falling sometimes, but at least no longer wallowing in the pit of inertia and self-pity. My journey back to myself had started, and I knew that with the proper focus, I could reach my goal of happiness and a full life.

In October '95, I returned to the University as a Sociology tutor, much to the excitement of the students concerned, some of whom I had taught in the past. I still remember the first class. It was not easy to face the roomful of faces from a wheelchair and I almost felt threatened by the students. When I took to the floor I could feel that I was not in balance, shaky and unsure of myself. I wanted to move around – back and forth and to the sides – the way I used to do. I guess I was missing those earlier teaching days of energetic jumping up and down, conducting my classes like a showman, with bursts of physical energy that propelled me on and off desks and across the lecture room floor; interacting with the class at close range and holding the attention of the students with my sheer exuberance. Now I was limited to strained arm movements at a distance. But I was not there to reminisce about my past way of doing things. My assignment was to lead a discussion around the policies of social transformation and their implications for labour relations in the private and public sector institutions of South Africa. I came well-prepared, having done my readings and consulted widely for 'wisdom'. I have never been one to cut corners with work. From the moment I uttered the first word, the old discipline took over and everything else was forgotten but the task at hand. I knew that this was an important first step, and that it had to be taken and accomplished well before I could move on. I didn't rush things but felt my way along slowly until I felt confident to delve more deeply into the core of the issues under discussion.

When we came to the subject of the Affirmative Action Policy, I tackled it by using the case of disability as an example.

'You cannot put disabled, wheelchair-bound athletes at the same starting line as able-bodied sprinters in a fast speed race and hope that they will all reach the finishing line simultaneously. The disabled athletes would naturally lose by far unless you positioned them strategically a few yards in front of the others, and equipped them with enough skill, knowledge and mind-power to race for the finish line from that point of "advantage". By giving them a head-start, you would have balanced the scales in the competition and equalised the possibilities of winning for all the athletes. Do you then call that "preferential treatment", or maybe . . . "reverse discrimination"? Because I don't!'

I still remember emphasising that point, directing my words particularly towards those in the class who felt that the policies of affirmative action are merely reversed discrimination in favour of blacks and against those perceived to have benefited from past rule. I noticed that the disability example seemed to open their eyes and make them less defensive about their positions.

I really enjoyed the rest of the class and was overwhelmed when, at the end, all the students got to their feet and clapped for me. It was a very moving moment. Then and there I vowed to myself that I would never fall so far down again. I also made a conscious resolution to love myself and erase that nagging sense of shame I carried with me. I was elated by my successful debut in the public arena, completely energised by the experience of being once again reunited with the crowd – my lifelong passion. I went home afterwards and thought about the seminar and the feelings it had evoked in me over and over again. The experience had taught me something about myself and my disability – that there is power to be found in what many might perceive as 'weakness', but that this power only shows itself if it is given the chance to flex its muscle. The disability example I had used in the seminar also opened my eyes to the fact that my disability was far from being just a negative burden; it had the capacity to change people's views about life and how they relate to each other. The first step on my long journey to recovery and rehabilitation had been taken. I knew that there were still many hurdles to surmount along the way. But at least I was on the right path. I had recovered that vital belief in myself, and my competitive streak that was so much a part of my vitality had been reawakened. In the competition called life, I was still a player in the game. With enough hard work, determination and incentive, I could still vault for that golden finish line along with the best of them. From that moment onwards, I never looked back.

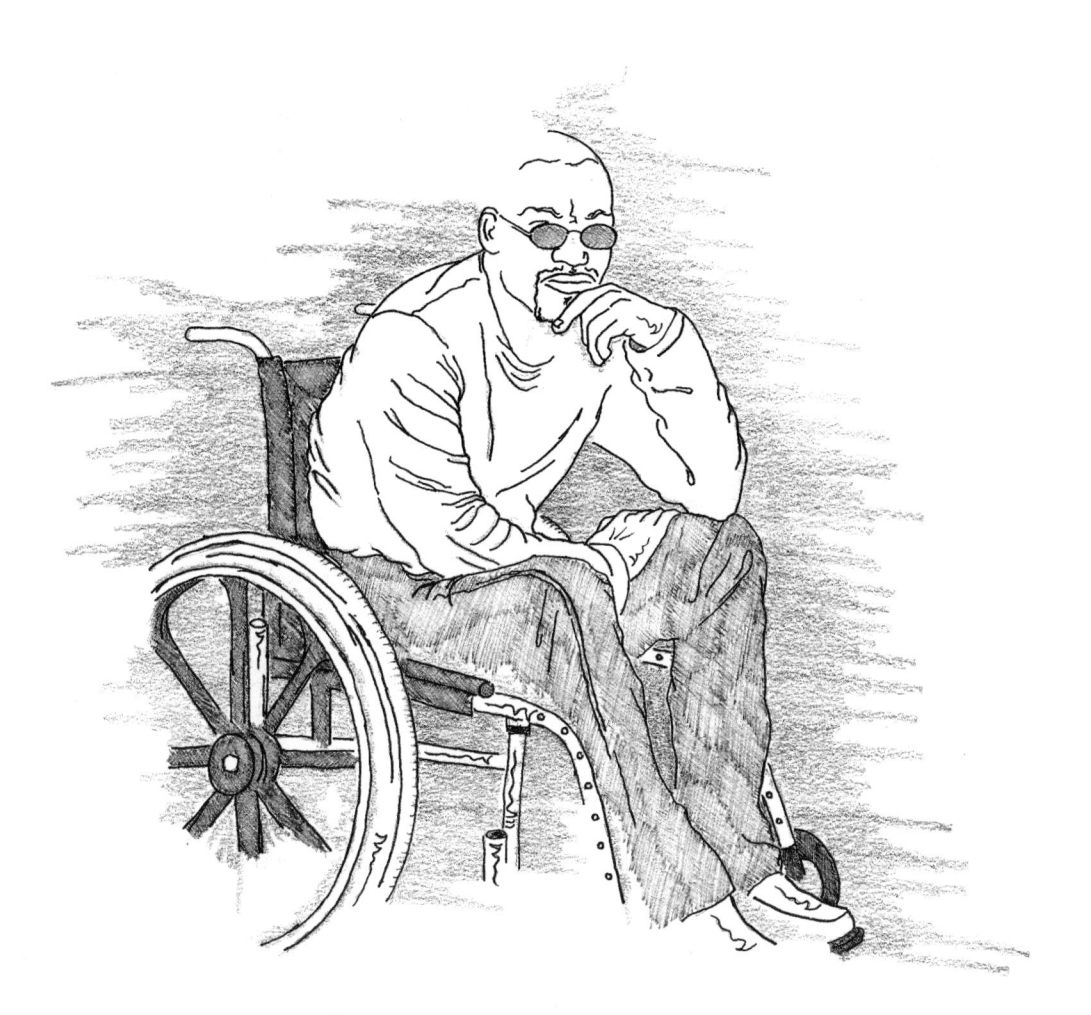

# Thisability

## *Dreams: You Make Them Happen*

You have to reach out and touch
Take that first step up the stairway
And make your move on the dance floor
To make your dreams come alive

It is your call to spark that flame for your fire
To kneel on the ground and blow so as to fan the blaze
To reach higher and light the lantern on the sidewalk
That will light up your path in this life of dreams and wishes

Only you can plan and execute your mission
And this takes a clear and steady vision
Do not allow yourself to be clouded by vain ambition
And do not ever forget, that crops are ready with the season

You must rise after each fall along your journey
Remember life is not a smooth sail on a quiet ocean
There will be storms and rumbles, darkness and the night
You need to be strong to survive the tests of your dreams

Dreams – you make them happen
But this is an art that is only mastered by hunters and explorers
Those that are ready to spread their wings and fly with the winds
This is not a game for those who wait for another day . . .

# 5

The year 1996 was a turning point in many ways. It got off to a good start, with me subjecting my body to a rigorous exercise programme that included aqua-therapy, reflexology and acupuncture. A good friend from my Mushroom days presented me with a homemade electric bicycle that exercised my legs, and day-in and day-out I was at it. It was a very simple machine, with no wheels, just electrically-driven pedals that you strapped your feet into. It gave me a very good work-out, which left my legs shooting with energy. Exercising also helped to promote my blood circulation, stimulate my central nervous system, keep my muscles flexible and my body active. Over time, all this hard work paid off, because I started to experience more sensations down my legs and, with this programme, also improved control over my bladder and bowels. The best part was when I woke up one morning to be confronted by a respectable morning erection – there he was standing, staring at me. I called everybody in the house to come and witness 'the miracle'. It had been ten months since my 'manhood' had last 'raised the flag'. With all these amazing improvements in my physical state, my confidence soared too. At times I tried too hard, and it only exhausted me. But my progress remained steady, even though the pace was slower than I sometimes would have liked. I even redeveloped my chest – every man's 'ego-box'. In the months immediately following my accident, I had acquired a strong fear of women, but with these new developments I felt at ease with the idea of going back to dating. Later, as I grew more confident in my sexual encounters, I started experimenting with new positions and styles. With all these heartening successes, my sorrows shifted to the back seat, and I tentatively began to 'flash my smiles' again.

The second quarter of '96 saw another milestone reached in my personal goals list. I went back to full-day work, employed as a contract researcher with Shell Livewire, a community outreach initiative intended to identify small business entrepreneurs and help them to develop their skills. It was exactly the right timing for me. I had regained enough confidence by this stage to be comfortable with being left alone, without my support system of brothers around me. I admit that the first few days in my new environment were a bit frightening, and I was grateful to be sharing my office not with a stranger, but with my employer – an old friend whom I knew well and could relate to very comfortably. She was beautiful, fashionable and quick-off-the-mark and, most important, she believed in me. This opportunity was a valuable stepping stone for me as it allowed me once again to exercise my initiative and exhibit my potential. She also paid me very well, which meant that I could be self-supporting. I will always be grateful to this good friend for allowing me the chance to prove myself again in a working environment – a chance that many who find themselves disabled are never given. This job was my springboard back into the public arena, where I could once again impress and express myself. It drew me closer to my core desire – to be reintegrated with others and listen to their stories as I told them mine. The people – 'the crowds', as I thought of them – were my world. I loved working with communities, and even before the crash, I had wanted to be an active participant in the processes that would help to advance my developing society to higher levels of self-actualisation.

My ability to deliver on the projects I became involved in stood me in good stead and it wasn't long before I was 'nabbed' by other consultants to assist with their development projects too. In no time, I was in demand as a tutor, researcher, field worker and presenter, at one stage fielding five jobs simultaneously. I badly needed the validation of a busy schedule. It allowed me to stay out late away from home, distracted me from the less savoury crowds I had started to hang out with, and kept me focused on what was positive and achievable.

In late '96, I joined forces with Vusi Ndimeni and a few other disabled friends and we formed a Support Group for the Disabled, based at the University of Durban-Westville and assisted by Rene Stewart, who headed the Occupational Therapy Department there. Up until then, I had avoided contact with other disabled people and I went only reluctantly, at Vusi's persuasion, to the first meeting. But once there, I soon saw what a powerful tool such a group could be in the common battles we all faced. We started visiting newly disabled 'patients' in hospitals, encouraging them to face and fight their pain. By then, I had come to realise that the only way I could come to accept myself and move on with my life, was by talking about my world and being with people who had lived through similar experiences. I had to open up and allow others to understand my pain, to be able to listen to them telling me that everything would be all right – and believe it. I still maintain that disability is not an easy condition to accept; it tears you apart. The Support Group was a brilliant idea as it allowed us to share our stories of pain as well as our victories. We played sport and discussed various disability-related themes. There were tears and laughter, silence and jubilation, questions and answers. I always felt relieved of my burdens when I was with the others in my group. I have become a strong advocate for such support initiatives and believe that they are a key component of healing and recovery, whatever the area of need or trauma. My group helped me through some important turning points. I made good friends and uncovered a lot of secrets about disability – knowledge that has assisted me in establishing a much more harmonious relationship with my 'Wheel Wagon'.

Most of the people with disabilities that we visited in the hospitals and homes reminded me of my own fears. Some of these fears I had already managed to allay, but others were still haunting me: 'Will I ever be able to walk again?' 'Am I ever going to be able to perform in bed and please my partner?' 'If I cannot ejaculate then where is the thrill and does this mean I will never father my own babies?' 'What if I wet my pants in public, what will people think of me?' 'What is the purpose to life now if I can't even go back to work and nurture my future?' 'Why me and what now?' Becoming disabled in adulthood leaves you with a lot of questions, especially in the beginning. It helps to have someone who can tell you what it all means and what to do when the going gets tough. I was fortunate in that I returned to a family who could meet my needs, answer my questions and promote my development. Others are not so lucky; for them, all the lights go out. They are left alone and isolated . . . locked into a world of their solitude and fears. Most are in need of a hero to inspire them, to be their symbol of hope and encouragement. Just as I was, they are searching for someone to tell them that everything is going to be all right. I would make friends with them and advise them to face their pain, to try and come to terms with their new condition as quickly as they could, and not wait until the inertia of despair had set in and it was too late to bounce back to life. I had learnt from my own situation the vital importance of recovering your spirit as early as possible. Hospital offers you safe space, a quiet time to think and assess and plan for what will come after. When you go home, you are faced with the harsh reality of just how much has changed in your world. By the time you are discharged, if you haven't already found your resolve and worked out your game plan, it will be much harder. Every time a 'patient' had doubts about the possibility of a happy future, I would remind him or her of the late Prof Friday Mavuso – the 'Chariot of Fire', as I chose to remember him. Friday was wheelchair-bound, yet in spirit, he was free. His strength and courage in fighting for the betterment of the disabled in South Africa transformed him into a hero for many. He died in June 1995, two months after my crash. How I wish he was still around! He gave meaning to human dignity and inspired many with his creed that 'it's not over until it's over'. All I attempt and achieve, I dedicate to him. He is the 'Chariot of Fire' because Friday on his wheelchair was in a fight for light. Wherever he is now, beyond the clouds, I hope he knows the depth of my gratitude for the lesson he taught me – to stand tall, no matter how bad the fall.

Our ailing world is in desperate need of inspiring role models, and inspiration resides with those who persevere and overcome. Friday was the embodiment of those qualities. I don't remember ever hearing about his educational qualifications – in fact, rumour has it that this Great Warrior of Wisdom never even reached Secondary School. However, in recognition of his role in uplifting the social status of people with disabilities, the University of Cape Town awarded him an Honorary Doctorate in Social Sciences. Friday recognised no limits to his own achievement or that of others, and his slogan was 'freedom and equity'. He was a natural-born leader with charisma and charm who was never afraid to make a stand on issues. Disability positioned Friday to exercise his influence on other people's destinies, not just the disabled, but society in general. He had a natural charisma and believed passionately in the causes that he espoused – one of them being his stance against township violence. Seeing him in action, you became so wrapped up in the energy of what he was saying that you would forget he was in a wheelchair.

1997 was another illuminating year for me. Together with my long-time friend Tobias and my younger cousin Q, I was employed by RUSU – the Rural and Urban Studies Unit at the University of Natal – to investigate the viability of community development co-operatives supported by private sector institutions as part of their social service initiatives. One of the areas we visited was Emseleni in northern KwaZulu-Natal, and it was here that I found real peace of mind and truly laid the ghosts of the past to rest. Two full years had passed since the crash that had left me paralysed, and all through that time, I was still holding onto the dream that my ability to walk – and with it my former life – would come around again. When we reached Emseleni, it was as if I finally closed the chapter and came to accept that my former life was gone for good. The whole environment at Emseleni took me back in time, reminding me of my past days as a boy with the TTT outreach programme. I found myself thinking of the long road distances we used to cover then, just as with the RUSU project of the present, and the 'brotherhood talks' that Q and I engaged in between the towns – because Q was always there with me, even back then. I thought of my times with Tobias at University and the dreams we shared of going out and working for the upliftment of our people in their developing communities. As I interacted with the workers at the site of one of the Emseleni co-operatives, I was reminded of the Human Resources development initiatives that were part of my duties at Tongaat Mushrooms. I found, as I relived each of these memories, that this act of revisiting was giving me the chance to pay my respects and then lay the past to rest. I realised that each of those goals and dreams of my past had come to fruition, had enriched me, made me wiser, and readied me to dream the new dreams of the future.

At Emseleni I discovered, as though for the first time, that even though I was in a wheelchair, I was still in the heart of the community. Nothing had really changed. My dreams were still attainable; all that was required was the effort and passion to reach for them and make them happen. It was time to move on with my life and not let the ghost of my former walking days keep me prisoner and sap my life-force. It was at Emseleni that I made a conscious decision to stop hiding behind my denials, to come to terms with the inescapable reality that I was paralysed, and accept without bitterness the changes this entailed.

In May 1998, my arrested career path regained its trajectory, and at the age of 26, I was appointed as the Director of the *Asiphephe* 'Let Us Be Safe' Road Safety Project – a sub-directorate within the KwaZulu-Natal Department of Transport. I went for the interview with a clear mind and a well-thought-out plan. As I sat waiting for my turn along with the other candidates, I had interesting thoughts going through my head. All of the other applicants were able-bodied. Far from feeling disadvantaged by this, however, I was convinced that I, with my disability, had a better story to tell and a good case to present. My reasoning was that no one can issue a sterner warning to others on the subject of road safety than someone who has tasted firsthand the damning consequences of road calamity. The preventative message of road safety is left incomplete if it does not also reflect the tangible consequences of disability and long-term pain that are the legacy of many individuals 'lucky enough' to survive a car crash. Crashes blind people, amputate their limbs, destroy their brains and maim them in many other terrible ways; a crash scars you for life. I, in my wheelchair, was living proof of the road safety message in a way that none of the other applicants could be. I also had no fear of facing the panel – to me, interviews are theatrical scenes where I get the chance to speak of my dreams and outline my plans to turn them into a reality that can be shared by all. When my turn came to go into the boardroom, I even jokingly asked the other applicants to phone me and congratulate me when the results were announced. I guess I was feeling specially confident that day – it was one of those days when everything seemed possible. And that was the aura I carried with me into the interview room.

The following evening, when the then Deputy Director General phoned me on my cellphone to inform me of my appointment, I simply laughed. I was with my brothers in the University park when the call came, and we celebrated with brotherly handshakes and outbursts of 'Yes!' – fists clenched in elated salute. The accident that, three years before, had foiled my ambitions to seize the Directorship of the Tongaat Huletts Human Resources Division had, in a strange twist, equipped me for a Directorship elsewhere; life is a mysterious series of cycles indeed! It was time to don my armour and ready myself to take my mission of disability into the very halls of government. In my mind, I saw this as a symbolic victory, the triumphant assertion of life over despair and defeat. This was my private revolution and by managing to stage a successful coup against the forces of disability, I felt that I could claim my rightful place in the Halls of Valhalla – where the brave Warriors of Scandinavian legend find their reward in happy eternity. I couldn't stop beaming as I broke the news to my family, who were all delighted for me. I was particularly ecstatic that I had achieved something momentous that rewarded all of them for their support and unwavering belief in me.

The *Asiphephe* Project is a government strategy aimed at reducing the high incidence of road crashes that has been the cause of far too many deaths and disability cases in the province of KwaZulu-Natal. The Project was designed to heighten awareness about the consequences and costs associated with irresponsible road user behaviour. KwaZulu-Natal alone loses an estimated R2 billion per annum as a result of road carnage – calculated in terms of lost manpower hours, the cost of emergency services, Road Accident Fund claims, insurance pay-outs and the like. And this figure runs parallel with the incalculable cost of the thousands of lives that are either lost or permanently destroyed. As Director of the Project, my job description was explicit: to oversee the co-ordinated implementation of Road Safety policy, strategies and programmes in KwaZulu-Natal. I was directly accountable to both the Minister of Transport and the public for my actions.

When I joined the KwaZulu-Natal Department of Transport I was struck by the fact that, as an institution, it had the capacity to support and promote the needs and interests of people with disabilities, both internally within its own units, and externally throughout KwaZulu-Natal. As a person in a wheelchair, I am very passionate about matters relating to disability and I felt it was one of my challenges to ensure that the Department's vision of 'Prosperity Through Mobility' also included disability issues. Although my job description did not specifically state that I was to be involved in disability matters, I did not see this as a problem. I went ahead anyway, initiating or participating in various activities that sought to develop better awareness of people with disabilities in our transforming society, and improved well-being and living standards for those affected. When our Minister acquired a donation of two wheelchairs from a local taxi association, he handed them over to me to present to the chosen candidates. I found a lot of pleasure in being a part of this uplifting occasion and witnessing the joy of the two young recipients. Knowing from my own experience the new lease on life that mobility can give, I was able to empathise from the heart with their elation. I was reminded of my own feelings all those years ago, when Vusi Ndimeni first initiated me into the secrets of hand control driving, reopening doors to the outside world and reuniting me with a part of my spirit that I thought I had lost forever. Mobility for a disabled person – whether in the form of a wheelchair or driving access – is a vital step to re-integration and self-actualisation.

The *Asiphephe* campaign went from strength to strength, gaining enormous popular support, attracting a range of stakeholders and continually refining its own strategies from the experiential lessons learnt. In 1998, the *Asiphephe* Focus Days held in the various developing communities of KZN to improve road safety awareness saw a major change in focus, as 'disability through road crashes' was introduced as the main theme. The exercise of changing human behaviour, particularly bad road user behaviour, sometimes calls for shock tactics, where the full extent of the possible consequences of the negative behaviour is driven home. This was the thrust of one of our more successful mass media strategies. Above all other things, people fear disability, and it is my belief that if given the choice, many would rather pass on from this world than face the suffering of a life without a limb, without sight or independent mobility. Most people still want to avert their eyes or close their ears in horror at the sight or mention of disability. The campaign was repeated during the following Easter period of 1999 where, as part of promoting the disability theme, *Asiphephe* prepared three mobile trailers, which carried a message to drive slowly and showed a man in a wheelchair with the message: 'I wonder if these new wheels can do 160 kph?' These mobile billboards were very well received by the public. Their message was strong and highlighted two realities, the first being disability and its everyday hardships, and the second, the fact that one of the major causes of disability is road crashes. People with disabilities were invited to the Focus Day events to tell their stories and add their experiences of struggle to the general emphasis, the intention being to send a strong message to all road users that the majority of road-accident-related disabilities are preventable. The campaigns also called on communities to assist and show understanding for those who were currently living with the consequences of serious injury resulting from road crashes.

The government White Paper on disability, the Integrated National Disability Study of 2000, states that: 'One of the greatest hurdles disabled people face when trying to access mainstream programmes is negative social attitudes. It is these attitudes that lead to the social exclusion and marginalisation of people with disabilities.' The *Asiphephe* Focus Days were partly aimed at combating these negative social attitudes, by allowing both able-bodied and disabled people to share common ground as part of the same campaigns and exchange experiences. It was a good exercise in that it gave people the chance to learn from each others' tragedies. Families with disabled members got the chance to walk around the various display stands and see what to do and who to contact in order to ease the complications that faced their loved ones at home and in society. People living with disabilities were given a platform to talk about their lives, share with others the hardship and fear of being isolated through their disabilities, and voice their dreams of being accepted by the wider society.

In July/August 1998, I visited the State of Victoria in Australia to see how they had dealt with their road accident problems – instituting measures that were successful to the point where they now have one of the lowest road death/crash records in the world. My mission was to learn from them and take their strategies and principles back for customised application in my own land. It was my first overseas experience and I was thrilled to have my first taste of it in a highly developed country like Australia. I took my cousin Maqkawe with me to share the experience. We visited Perth, where we landed after our direct flight from Johannesburg, stayed and worked in Melbourne, and had a brief stint in Sydney. We met a few fellow South Africans who had left this country in the late 70s to escape political persecution and made some friends – among them some Sudanese cab drivers, who were interested to know more about South African luminaries such as former President Nelson Mandela, the Archbishop Desmond Tutu and our local Reggae star, Lucky Dube. Hey! These brothers from worlds far away knew about and admired my countrymen – I felt very proud to be a South African child. We toured Melbourne and participated in a few Road Safety exercises with the officers from the local Traffic Department – just to observe and learn. It was a life-changing experience in many ways, one that broke a few personal barriers for me. I had been on an aeroplane before, but I had never imagined that overseas travel was still possible for me now that I was in a wheelchair. Yet here I was, paralysed, and enacting the unthinkable dream. And what was more, enacting it because of, not in spite of, my paralysis, since it was that very disability that had brought the experience into my orbit.

While in Australia, I also made time to meet with different disability organisations to learn about how they had assisted their government in meeting the needs of disabled Australians. Australia is an extremely well-developed society that has implemented proactive measures to cater for the needs of all its citizens – including those who are disabled. I learnt a lot from my time in this country and was fascinated by their disability-friendly infrastructure, including some of their social programmes that actively encourage the participation and leadership role of people with disabilities. Their public transport systems, their rehabilitation facilities, their housing policy – even their telephone booths – are designed for equal use and access. Theirs is one of the most impressive re-integration models that I have witnessed. The success of it was visible in the eyes of most of the people with disabilities that I met – you could see their optimism, despite their limitations. I wished for the same opportunities for my own people back home.

My Australian visit left me with a lot of food for thought, especially in the area of disability re-integration, in that it provided fresh input into common problems and allowed me to see, first-hand, possibilities that worked. Soon after my return, I was involved in a project to establish accessible public transport systems for people with disabilities – something I considered of vital importance. It is well-known that one of the major hurdles that hinders the process of the re-integration of people with disabilities into mainstream society is the absence of adequate transport facilities. What was particularly gratifying about this new project was that it was a KwaZulu-Natal Department of Transport assignment that required the involvement of all disability stakeholders in its planning, implementation and monitoring. The final result was the distribution of three buses specially designed to meet the needs of disabled passengers. I was ecstatic when the buses were introduced into KwaZulu-Natal because this marked a turning point in both attitude and approach to issues of disability in this country. For the first time, the provision of transport required not just the mapping out of bus routes, but doing in-depth research into the areas where the disabled were located. It was also a first for South Africa in that it required a different approach to the engineering of the buses, in the sense of having to equip a moving vehicle with a hydraulic lift.

Two of these buses have been circulated in urban disadvantaged communities – 'the harbours of disabled wrecks', as I refer to these townships, since these are the areas where, all too often, black disabled people become stranded, stagnating in their forgotten corners with no access to any of the vital currents of opportunity. The third bus operates within Durban's city centre and caters for a wider constituency of not only disabled passengers, but the aged and infirm. Each of the buses is equipped with a hydraulic lift that provides easy and independent access for wheelchair-bound passengers. These measures were not only designed to provide the disabled with independent access to transport, but to restore their dignity, along with their sense of belonging and independence. Our society is poorly-equipped in terms of services and infrastructure that would allow disabled people to integrate and participate in economic and social activities. As a result, people with disabilities are always left behind on the sidewalk. This not only imprisons them literally, but inhibits their potential, leaving them without hope of improvement. The Department's support of this 'accessible transport' project has put in place an infrastructure of inestimable value for the communities concerned and done much to aid the empowerment of the disabled in those areas.

I was very honoured when I was approached and asked to give the buses a name. I proposed the name '*Sukuma*', which in English translates to 'stand up and rise' – and was delighted when my suggestion was accepted. The buses are painted yellow – the colour of light, symbolising hope. I have already said how disability steals away an individual's sense of independence and keeps many locked away behind the doors of their homes; to me, the buses were symbolic of a break-out from this prison of hopelessness. The road is a vital tool for rehabilitation, and my own experience has been that travelling and seeing the world frees the mind from its entrapping walls of self-pity and dependency. I felt that the name given to the buses should express this sense of freedom.

The three *Sukumas* were officially launched by the MEC of KZN Transport at a joyful ceremony in December 1998, attended by disabled people from a range of different ages and backgrounds. I subsequently had the pleasure of personally unveiling one of these buses to the selected community at a celebration in Durban which formed part of International Day for People Living with Disabilities. I enjoyed every minute of this experience and went away greatly inspired, particularly by the strength of character shown by the many young people with disabilities, who participated enthusiastically in the celebrations with a talented display of poetry, story telling, dance, music, drama and art. The community were thrilled by the sight of a bus that had been specifically designed for them and all scrambled to be among the first to go on board, those on wheelchairs mounting on the hydraulic lift. I am not one to cry in public, but on that day I could feel the burning tears behind my lids. To me, the road is life itself, and the motion of driving is like the blood of vitality coursing through the veins. I knew that for these people, the journey out of stagnation had started; through the mobility of transport, they were being freed from their forgotten corners, reconnected to the world and all its possibilities. Research surveys that have since been conducted to evaluate the effectiveness of the initiative indicate that the disabled and aged of all races in the pilot communities are making the most of the resource they have been given. It still gives me a warm feeling to this day whenever I happen to see one of 'our' sunshine yellow *Sukuma* buses passing by.

## *I Almost Wished (For Yesterday)*

I almost wished I could start all over again
Go back to my first day and draw my first breath
To my early months and attempt my first steps
To my childhood era and make new friends
Back to my golden teens and establish new interests
– a new life

I almost wished all of this was just a dream
That I would wake up and discover I was still young
With a life ahead and choices to explore
With time and opportunity to plan without mistake
And a chance to do all of this much better
– much wiser

I almost wished I had not yet loved at all
That I was still out there in search of the perfect woman
That she was in my dreams and still to meet me
Waiting for me to reach out and touch her
Waiting to step out of a crowd and dance with me
– swing with me

I almost wished someone could hold me tight
Tell me life is kind and that mistakes are forgiven
Tell me there is no need to look back and regret
Make me understand that tomorrow is still mine
Talk to me, take away my fears, show me the way
– saying all will be all right

I almost wished I had not come here
But now I know that I should not wish so
For it is with coming here that I have come to know
That yesterday was a journey where I discovered myself
And that every day was a good lesson that only grew me
– life goes on

I now only want to face my today
And keep my wishes for my tomorrow
For yesterday came to be, was
– and is gone . . .

# 6

My three year contract as Director of the *Asiphephe* Project came to an end in May 2001. I bowed out with pride, aware that during my term of office a solid foundation had been built for road safety awareness, with good accident reduction achieved. I was delighted when the Department extended my contract by another year, this time round as a Community Outreach Manager. My new portfolio involved a lot more travelling, since I was responsible for establishing and training Community Road Safety Councils – a vehicle through which the government aimed to take Road Safety programmes, infrastructure and equipment out to the developing areas of the province. I enjoyed the new position. It was the kind of job that came naturally to me, putting my people skills to good use, and once again I felt that my wheelchair added a special impact to the message I was imparting. I established wonderful relationships with the communities that I worked with, and they made me even more determined to establish disability as an equal, not inferior, segment of our multi-faceted reality – just another shade in the spectrum of our beautiful diversity.

Since my accident, I have been presented with a lot of opportunities to share my story publicly, appearing in various arenas to talk and raise awareness around disability and its needs. It is my strong belief that many of these needs *can* be met by any society that heeds the inner voice of compassion and commits itself to this end. This entails persuading communities, government and business institutions to work together to assist with the social re-integration and economic upliftment of people with disabilities. There is still so much work to be done in this area – research on disability needs and location, awareness campaigns, improved social security and employment opportunities, development of adequate building infrastructure and transport systems and, last but not least, the implementation of counselling and rehabilitation systems geared to assist disabled people with their holistic re-integration into our society. It was always a source of great satisfaction to me that through the resources of the KZN Department of Transport, we were able to start redressing some of these lacks. The Department was always very receptive to my input and incorporated many of my proposals into its mainstream policy and activities. One of the areas we were able to focus on as a Roads Department was to promote awareness of the rights of road crash survivors and the resources they could access. Through structures like the Community Road Safety Councils and Rural Road Transport Forums, we instituted outreach programmes in developing communities aimed at educating disabled road crash victims about their right to compensation from the Road Accident Fund, and how to go about claiming from it. I consider myself fortunate to be living in a society that is so enlightened in these respects. However, the good intentions behind such initiatives are too often sabotaged by the legal 'vultures' – those unscrupulous individuals who use such funds for their personal enrichment at the expense of unsuspecting and vulnerable victims. In 1999, when the National Department of Transport indicated that it was to conduct an investigation into corruption and fraud with regard to the payment of compensation to road accident victims, it was the law associations that threatened to take the government to court for 'intruding into the privacy of their practices and affairs'. I am always at a loss to understand how someone can live a happy life of luxury knowing that they have taken from those in need, who are then left languishing in misery and pain. It is my strong belief that we need to come together as a society and take collective responsibility for ensuring that those who need it most are properly assisted and protected from the unscrupulous. I feel fortunate to have been able to work in environments that allowed me to exercise my social responsibility conscience, within institutions that shared my own concerns.

Experiences change us; our way of being and our identity, our views about life and our sense of purpose, the language we use to express what we are as well as the story we have to tell to the world. Tragedies take away from us, but they also present us with new opportunities and abilities. The 20th of April 1995 was the day my life altered forever. Along with the other changes it brought, the car crash forced me to reassess the way I viewed both myself and life in general. It made me grateful to be alive and presented me with the opportunity to be acquainted with my real purpose on this Earth. It forced me to write a different life story from the one of my early ambitions, allowed me to rediscover that I am an integral part of the human family, and not just an independent and self-serving individual. Up until the moment of the crash, I had lived a charmed life, one that lacked for nothing and was fortunate in every way. It was a life almost completely free of pain and restrictions. But life is not only about ourselves and our personal ambitions; it is about the humanity we share with others, and it is in service to that bond that we rediscover and heal ourselves. Disability has opened my eyes not only to the pain of others, but to my own internal prejudices towards the disabled, conditioned into me by the society I live in. My sole ambition now is to be an instrument of change, to use my experiences and talents in service of the struggle for the emancipation and dignity of all disabled South Africans. It is my burning wish to reach out to as many in need as possible, in the hope that my story will inspire others to find their own happy endings to the personal dramas of pain and trauma that hold them prisoner. As much as I believe that government and business have a crucial role to play in helping to elevate the status of disabled people in our society, I also feel strongly that, as with all struggles, it is those who are directly affected who need to take responsibility for leading their own march towards freedom, empowerment and visibility. This is how I choose to contribute towards the struggle for the recognition of people with disabilities – by writing a book and talking about my life, tracing the ups and downs that came with my experiences – and celebrating my changes as a sign of rebirth, not a mark of death.

When the new millennium dawned, it heralded in many ways my own 'new century'. The positive trends of the previous years had done a lot to boost my confidence. I had achieved some valuable goals in personal as well as professional terms and crossed a number of important hurdles. But in terms of 'life dreams', the year 2000 made those successes pale by comparison; this was the year that my 'rocket of fame' was really launched. One of the early highlights occurred in April, at the inception of the 2000 Road Safety Campaign 'Road Show'. This was a very ambitious programme, entailing a series of huge public gatherings scheduled for the different regions of the province as part of the awareness drive. The first 'show' kicked off during the Easter weekend, at the King Zwelithini Stadium in Umlazi, Durban. A crowd of close to 45 000 worshippers had gathered at the venue to pray for road safety as part of the Easter observance, and I was invited there to give a talk on road safety and the need for society to be accepting of difference and disability. Needless to say, I had accepted the invitation with alacrity. It is hard to describe the emotion I felt when I got out in front of the huge audience. My whole body shook with energy and elation. This was the chance that I had fantasised about my whole life – to stand out in front of an enormous crowd and hold them in the palm of my hand. I spoke from the heart, relating my story just as it came. The response overwhelmed me. As I finished, the huge crowd cheered and rose to its feet – an indescribable moment. I was 'in concert', just as I had always dreamed of being, performing 'myself' for a huge audience – *'ASIPHEPHE!'*

That 'moment of fame' sparked my career as a motivational celebrity. Many of those in the audience contacted me later with requests for more public appearances, to be the master of ceremonies or guest speaker at this or that upcoming family or social function. Then the calls started coming from magazines, who wanted to interview me or have me write the story of my life: *Cheers*, *Genuine*, *Drum* and others. I not only agreed to tell my story, but extracted a promise from them that they would henceforth make it their policy to feature others living with disability, who also had inspirational stories to tell. I got a lot of positive feedback from people coming forward to tell me that my story had taught them so much and requesting to visit me at home to continue the exchange. The momentum continued, and in June 2000, I was honoured to discover that the story of my life and my struggle with disability – which had appeared in *Drum* along with the interview they did on me – had been featured by the Department of Education as a chapter in a book titled *Kuyasa – Incwadi Yabafundi* (*It Is Dawning – A Book For Learners*), a motivational text aimed at Grade Eight in KwaZulu-Natal schools. It was humbling and exciting news – and I was over the moon. I felt that all the years of hard struggle were vindicated. Through the triumph my life had become, I had truly proven to the world that there is indeed 'Life After The Storm'. Remembering my own school days and how much I had enjoyed reading the stories of others' inspiring lives, I was particularly glad to know that this time round it was me who was being read about in the classrooms.

In October 2000, I was still riding the crest of the wave. What makes this month very special to me is the fact that it was during this time that I finally got to live out my longheld dream of recording a song. This song was part of the Road Safety awareness mission and its title was: *'Asiphephe, Let us be Safe'*. It was produced by Jabu Khanyile, one of South Africa's top musicians and a personal favourite of mine. My brothers and I were invited to participate in the shooting of the video version, in the company of other local artists who had been invited by Khanyile to take part. The video was put together by an amazing team at the South African Broadcasting Corporation studio in Johannesburg, and the result was a great success. It was flighted on national television throughout the 2000 festive season – a period inevitably associated with high numbers of crash incidents. The song itself, with its catchy tune, was very well received by communities as both a message and joyous melody, and it brought people together to shout a common slogan – *'Qaphela, Qalaza!'*, meaning: 'Be careful, look before you cross.' It made it to the top of the charts in some of the popular radio stations in South Africa, and also received coverage in other neighbouring countries; it was even shown on CNN. There I was on national television in my wheelchair, singing along and dancing away!

Hardly had the dust settled from that excitement, when I received a phone call from Neville Herrington of Thekweni Television Productions, who told me they were wanting to shoot a documentary of my life, to be flighted on a programme called 'Expressions' on SABC 3 later in the year. I was completely blown away with excitement when I heard this. I subsequently met with the film crew to map out how the documentary would go and which areas of my life it would focus on. They wanted it all – my childhood, my family, my educational and employment backgrounds, and of course, the changes I had been through in disability; the book I was working on, my poetry and drawings . . . everything, right down to my love for cars, my reflections on life, my dreams and future plans. They also interviewed my father, brothers, sisters and closest friends. I was given the chance to read some of my poems on camera, and was also filmed while drawing one of my sketches. I was thrilled by the whole experience – in my wildest dreams I could never have imagined that I would end up starring in my own life's movie! The very next week, *Tribute* magazine called, wanting to feature me in a special issue targeting high achievers and figures of status – the movers and shakers, dreamers and go-getters of our South African society. This was another unexpected accolade, one which signalled to me that in the public world, I had 'arrived' in style!

The first words that my father spoke to me all those years ago when he saw me lying crushed and broken on that cold hospital bed were: 'All things happen for a purpose.' I did not know what he meant then. But today, many years after the crash, I understand. It has taken me a long time to come to terms with what happened to me, but I can genuinely say that I am now happy and at peace with the fact that I have found a home in disability. There are still times when I ask myself if this had to happen to me at all. But I know that it did. It was God's Will, part of His Master Plan, and thus an episode in the story of my life that had to come to pass. During my time in hospital, one of my visitors was a young disabled street-kid called Joseph, whom I had befriended during my visits to the city centre. He was a boy of fiercely independent spirit, who used to wheel himself about on a skateboard. After he saw me in hospital, his words to my father were: 'I am happy that this one has been disabled. We need someone like him.' At the time, his words seemed very harsh to me. But I have come to see them in a different light, and to realise that my call to disability was a call to arms in service of a cause that badly needs its champions. Through it, so much has been unveiled to my eyes. I have come to appreciate the power of prayer and have been drawn closer to God and the peaceful acceptance of life and whatever it brings. I see myself now as an instrument of God's song – of His beautiful music of love and healing – and I 'sing' His message to the world in every way that I can.

Paralysis has cast a little more magic on me and offered me the chance for a new beginning. I have grown and matured enormously as a result of the accident. There are, of course, still times when I stumble and fall, when I break my head open trying to find answers where none exist. There have also been times when I have slipped off the path and resorted to self-destructive means to escape my prison. Then I have to make a special effort to be positive and patient with myself . . . and focus not on the fall, but on rising again. It's been a long, tough road to healing, filled with its share of setbacks, breakthroughs, challenges and triumphs – but I know that things are going to be okay for me now. I have found acceptance of what happened to me, and this has enabled me to embark on a whole new start.

Looking back over everything that has happened to me over the seven year span that this book recounts, I have to say that life has been kind to me and given me some of the best moments that a soul can ever wish to experience in this lifetime – I have almost had it all. As someone who loves the spotlight, I have been given many wonderful chances to take centre stage and perform the music that is me. And I have no doubt that many more of such rich and fulfilling moments lie ahead of me.

These days I have a lot of blessings to count. I am free from pain, in love and married to a wonderful woman who has restored to me a lost part of myself and inspired me to be able to love again and find truth and meaning in life. As I write these words, my cup of happiness is overflowing – for I have just become a father! My beautiful baby daughter, Swazi Tando-Lena Zulu, was born in McCord's Hospital in Durban on the 16th of April 2003. There are no words to describe the joy and gratitude I feel for this perfect little bundle of life that I hold in my arms – and for the miracle of fatherhood that has been granted to me.

If I could be given the chance to have my old life back, would I take it? Would I change the life I have now for the one that was? I don't ask myself those questions anymore. My only wish now is to embrace today, for tomorrow will come in its own way and yesterday has already been and gone.

# Part Two

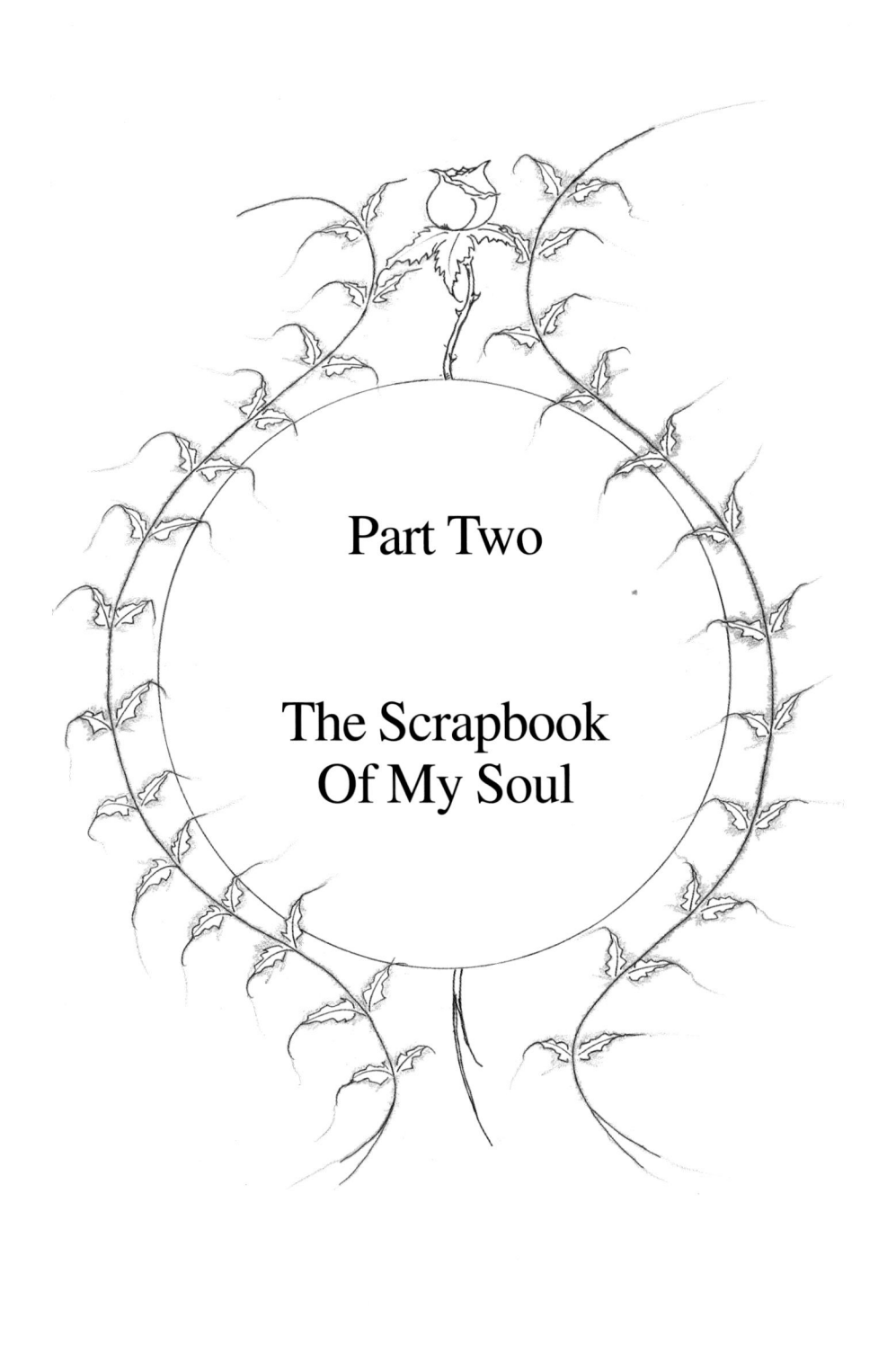

# The Scrapbook
# Of My Soul

# Crusader On Wheels

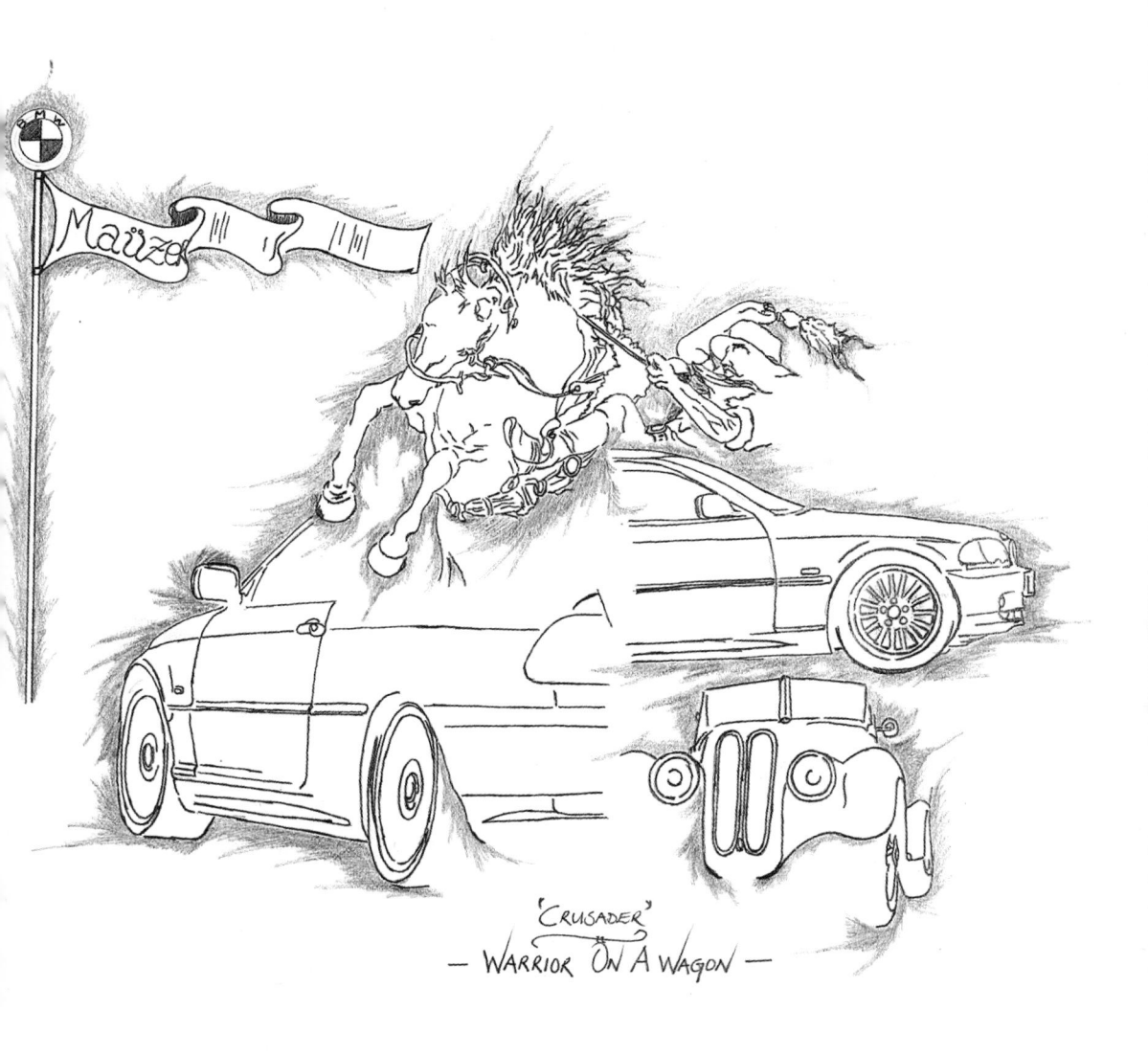

## *Crusader On A Wagon*

I have a Wish
I am driven by a Goal
A Mission that carries my Vision
This is my life's Purpose
I am a Crusader on a Wagon

I am speaking straight from my heart's parlour
My message is in words coated in colour
I am saying to you that the spice of life is diversity
Why then in difference do we tend to spark the flames of adversity?
Who is it that said we are different and thus unequal in potential?
I remind you that in God's eyes even those who are invisible are special

I am saying do not close your eyes and say *I* am blind
Do not fail to understand and laugh at me saying I am out of my mind
Who said I can reach the end of the line only if I walk
I will fall and rise, stutter through my words and finally talk
I am a child of the earth and believe me it is you who has fears
I grow stronger every time you notice me and you silence your jeers

I am saying to the world that you are all fathers and brothers
That these others are your children, your sisters and your mothers
With disregard we have built prisons where children cannot write on the walls
Loneliness can never be the stairway of hope that we climb over the falls
How can these broken wings help me reach out and touch a saving hand
If no one is nowhere around to see to my needs and that they mend?

I always believed there was nothing impossible about conquering Mars
I say to you all souls can shine in the skies like the brightest stars
That every child is born with a gift to spread their wings and impress
My message says they all can if only allowed the pride to express
I have chosen to travel the open road – for this I was born
For this message cannot be delivered by those who are airborne

I have a wish that every child lives a full life to eternity
I am driven to speak to all of you by a beautiful goal of equity
I have covered miles on a journey to build my mission
That will unite the world around a shared and noble vision
This is my life's purpose that I happened to stumble upon
I am a messenger – a Crusader on a Wagon . . .

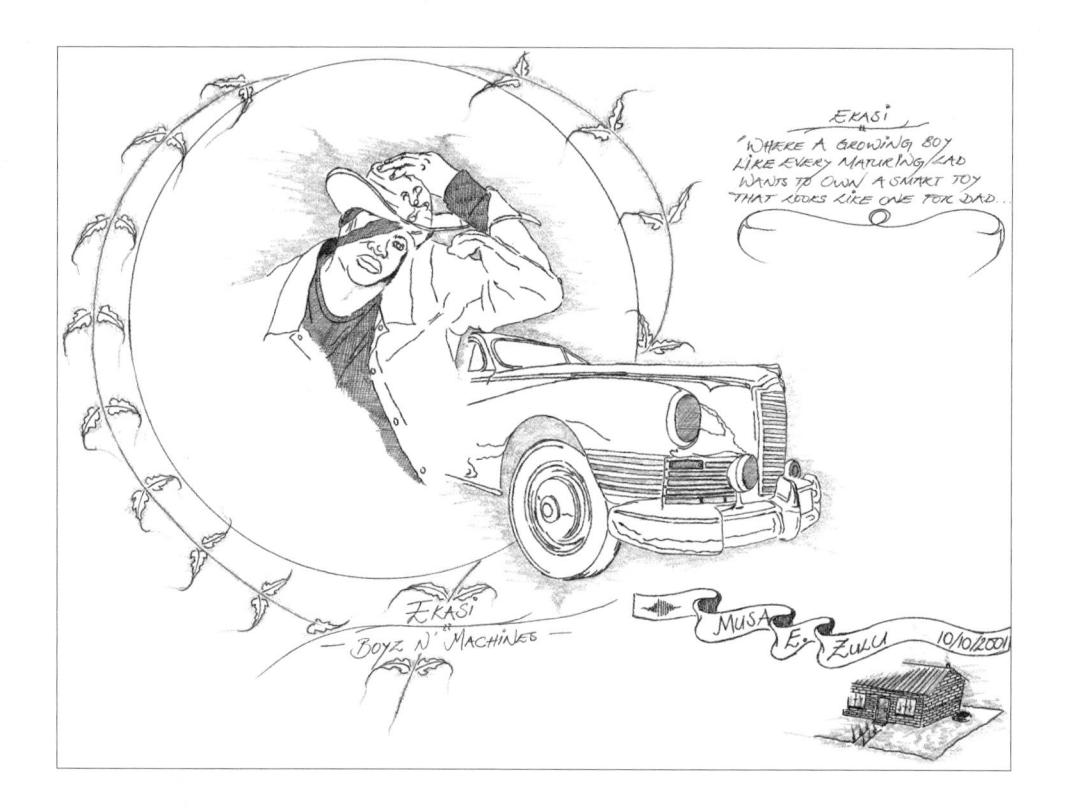

My interest in cars started at an early age. As a young boy I loved toy cars, and mine were always altered to express the exact look I wanted. I couldn't wait to grow up and drive. My driving career began with bricks in the sand and progressed to remote controlled miniatures. To me, driving was a symbol of utmost pleasure, power and independence. When we were young boys in our teens, our bedroom wall was a mosaic of Ferraris, Porsches and Lamborghinis – Boys and Machines. We had plenty of toys and played with them together from dusk till dawn. My brothers and I loved our cars with passion, and I knew even as a child that I was never going to settle for anything less than perfect wheels when I grew up. I loved sitting beside my Old Man when he drove, getting enormous pleasure from watching him turning the wheel, taking the corners, overtaking other cars and changing gears. It seemed a very macho activity to me, the thing that men do.

**B**MW is 'my car', my special passion. To me, the BMW design is the epitome of automobile aesthetics, the ultimate expression of human technological innovation and excellence. I have been very fortunate to have been allowed by Forsdicks – the BMW manufacturer in South Africa – to 'create' my own custom-altered versions of models I have bought from them. This has enabled me to live out my fantasy of Big Boys' Toys. In the last six years, my 'collection' has included 'Bulldogs and Tigers', 'Green Mambas and Panthers', 'Haunting Shades and Desert Sands'. Each of these cars reflected a different stage of my journey to recovery and acceptance, outer expressions of my mood and emotions of the time. All were either converted to or came with automatic gearbox, with specially adapted hand controls around the steering wheel for accelerating and braking. This means that I use my hands to drive, and I have come to enjoy 'pushing' my cabs along in this way; for me it represents the driving experience in its purest form. This system of driving has also helped me to develop my arm muscles and a chest 'box', which in turn has contributed to my regaining balance and control over my posture. So my BMWs have played an integral role in my rehabilitation. I call them my 'Mauzers' – the Mauzer being the First World War German gun of legendary reputation – in honour of my father, who earned the nickname for his performance on the tennis court. He was known for his power and precision, his blistering forehand strokes and devastating first serve. I love the smile it always brings to my father's face to see 'his name' engraved on one of his son's cars.

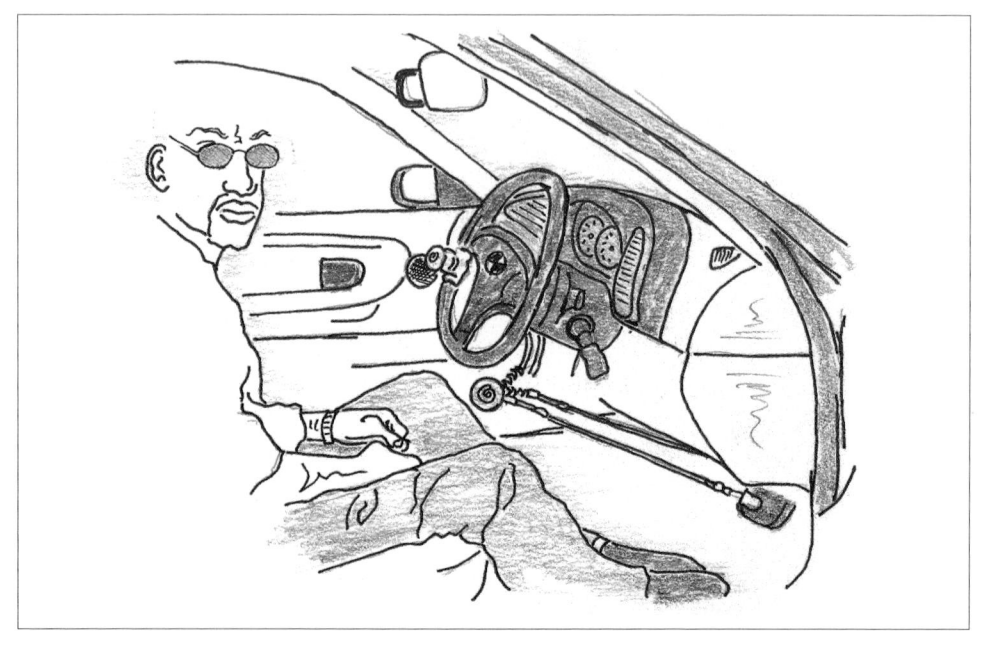

**HAND CONTROLS**

My cars are much more than simply 'wheels' to me; they are part of my 'language' of being – tangible expressions of the self I am and the world I live in. It is through them, their power and the mobility they make possible that I come to experience the beauty inside myself and the will to fulfil my dreams. My cars are a part of me, and that is even more the case now that I can no longer walk with my own legs – my cars 'walk' me. They do more than simply compensate for my loss, for it is when I am at the wheel and travelling the freedom of the limitless road that my spirit is set free. I am never more truly myself than when cruising to the music of my favourite songs and feeling my sense of connection to the beautiful world.

With each of the BMWs that I have 'created', owned and driven, I have learned to express myself and my state of mind better. Their custom-made designs are the 'melodies' we sing together as we travel the road of mobility and life. Their particular shapes, special features and chosen colour combinations have corresponded with the changing seasons in my own being – red and angry, humble and understated, powerful and predatory, confident and self-assured. My cars truly inspire and evoke 'The Language Of Me', for as they communicate with me through the 'songs' of mobility, I am moved to respond with the poetry of reflection. Many of the poems I have written were inspired by the feeling that bathes my soul while I am driving – or even just sitting – inside my cars. For this reason, I refer to my BMWs as . . . 'Bullets Of My Emotions'.

## *Bullets Of My Emotions*

Evolution, revolution
Red with anger
Aggressive to the core
Trapped in a need for recognition
You were my shooting star – GUSHESHE!
Every mother's worst nightmare
A dream from the days of my youth

Yet when I found you I cruised in a cold dream
Dead with the living in broad daylight
A shadow of a ghost in the darkness of the night
Wishing in silence for a moment of change
But pretending it's no big deal
I was going through the lessons of life . . .

Seasons change – green leaves, sand and a flash of lightning
Blending colours with nature, finding beauty in the dark
Down to earth, humbled by a new beginning
Peace and a warm home – my only burning feeling
'I'm still my father's child' – so said the song
I have realised all my desires in your gentle embrace
MAUZER, you found me my lost self

I am waltzing away in slow motion
One moment I am a dolphin swimming away
The next I am dancing to the strings of a symphony in G
Enjoying the power and pleasure of change
Blooming with the summer and warming up in winter
I come to life with every forest in the reaching mountain
Every plain, every cloud and every stream reflecting my colours . . .

I am pushing the wind with hand power
Riding the storm out
Not much today can stop me along my journey
Inside that cockpit lives the best of me
I am destined for Heaven in a spectrum of shades
In the colours of beauty and style – I am a chameleon
Pain can change itself to passion

I am learning from life and giving back a thing or two
Challenging the limit of the skies
Wiping the tears away for a smile
My prayer is that I will find life through my changes
And that with each mile I am drawn closer to God
Closer than ever before . . .

In the course of rehabilitating my sense of confidence and promoting my reintegration into society, my BMWs have also promoted a strong bond between myself and my 'other wagon' – my wheelchair. My BMW allows me to transfer to and from my wheelchair with pride and dignity; over time, I have come to feel very natural with the transfer and accomplish it smoothly. But for others less used to the event, it can sometimes be a startling transition. 'The Unbelievable!' is what a good friend and former work colleague – 'Master Mntungwa' – once christened me, in reference to the disbelieving expression on the face of an old man at a petrol station as he watched me climb out of the BMW to pay a visit to 'the small room' there. After seven years of being with me through thick and thin, across the range from 'iMatchbox' to 'iDolphin' and 'iG-String', over the hills and far away, my 'wheels of steel' have taken strain – but they are still going strong.

When my wheelchair first came into my life, its colour was pink, because I needed one in a colour that I hated – one that I would be determined to escape. But as time passed, I repainted it green to match the green BMW that I was driving then – the colour of acceptance. I will soon have to come to terms with the fact that a new wheelchair has to now step in and take me further. But I will miss this old wagon when that moment of parting finally comes; we have come to know and understand each other very well through the years. I discovered in a moment of reflection that I had actually grown fond of the 'object' and come to accept and cherish its presence and meaning over the years of my disability. I love my 'wheels of steel'; they define me, they tell my story and carry my message. My wheelchair is symbolic of my continuity, my search for purpose and my quest for completeness. If anybody were to forget to mention my wheelchair when they were introducing me to an audience, I would never respond to the call to come out to the front – for they would not have called out my full name. My 'wheelchair wagon', like my cars, is an integral part of my independence, belonging and mobility, and I just couldn't imagine my life without it.

THE LANGUAGE OF ME

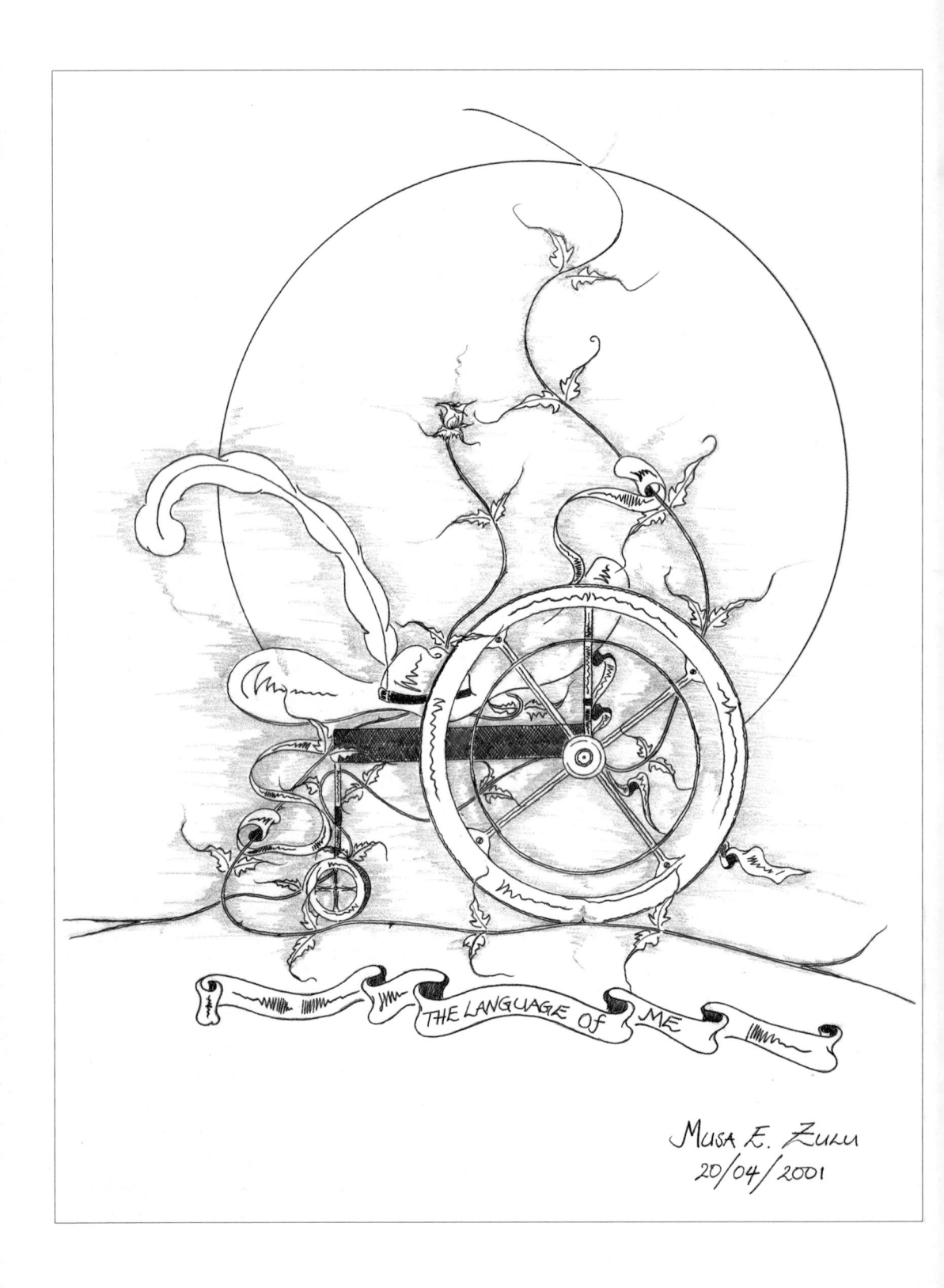

Musa E. Zulu
20/04/2001

## *These Wheels Of Steel*

I have at times during the past days wondered
What and where my life would be today
Had this tragedy of disability not met me
Leaving me confined to these wheels of steel

Maybe I would be walking up and down
Running around kicking balls with the boys
Maybe I would be jumping up high
To the beat of a song and its pounding drums
Maybe I would be climbing mountains
And scaling the walls to unexplored heights

Or maybe I would be dead . . .

Then I start to ponder and I discover
That on these wheels of steel I do move up and down
Sitting around and talking about the stories of peace and love
Doing things that lovers do – the things that you and I do
On these wheels of steel I still do jump up and down
Happy with the memories of having been a boy and now a man
I still dance to the songs and move with the beat and the drum
In my mind and life climbing mountains and scaling the walls
Exploring each height with every opportunity given

Yes, I have often wondered
When I sit down alone to think in quiet
Whether at all I do still wish for those maybes
And deep in my mind, body and soul I feel it
– Oh yes and this I do believe! –
That I really don't have any reason to regret
For all that I have ever wished for myself to be
Today I am
And every night before I fall asleep
I know I am glad to be alive
And about that – there is no maybe . . .

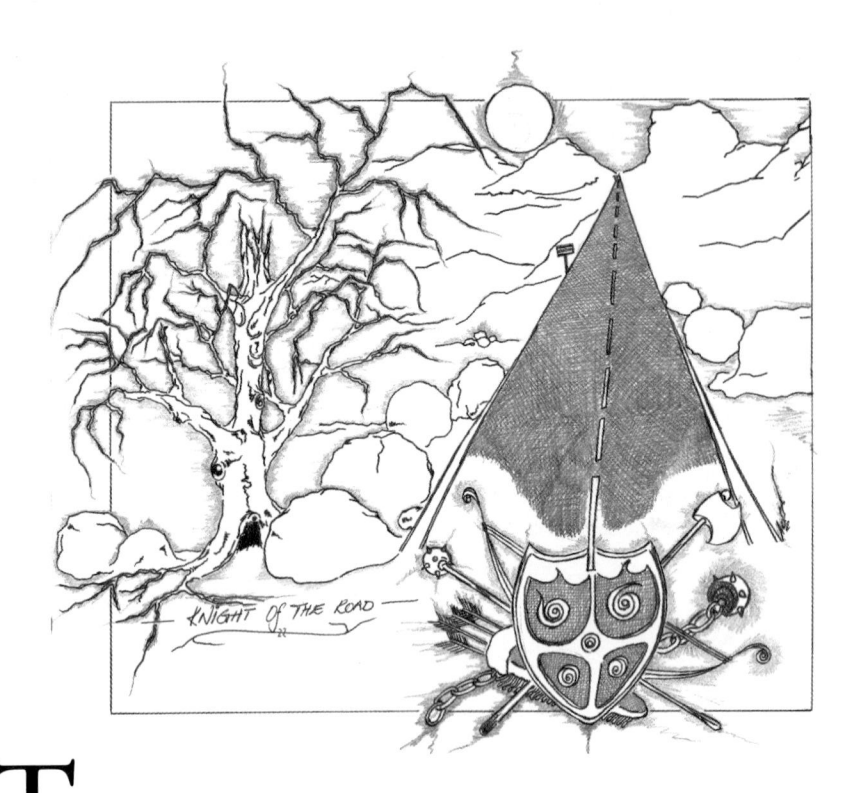

Throughout my working life, I have made it a point that the job opportunities I explored would allow me to inhabit my 'three favourite worlds' – on the road, at the wheel of a car, and heading for the destination of an audience. 'Outreach' has always been my first consideration before signing any employment contract; I know I would never be happy in the confined setting of an office. My fantasy is to be a Viking hero, and the road is, for me, the natural element of such heroes. I jump with joy inside when an appointment calls for me to drive to a place far away. There is an adventure in journeys, an unpredictability that calls forth my crusading spirit. I believe it is my mission to be out on the road and to show the world that a person with a disability *can* live a full life. When I step out of the car into my wheelchair, it is much more than a mere action – to me it is a statement. I am saying to the world 'look at me and see, listen and know – there is life everywhere, and it is up to all of us to help one another to find it and enjoy it to the best of our potential, desires and dreams'. It is people – my family, friends and strangers – who have helped me to climb the steps of hope and realise my potential, and I believe there are many others who could similarly transcend their pain if all of us extended the same helping hand to them. When I go out on my visits to various communities, I remind people of this precious lesson. I repeat it to children in schools and young people with disabilities in hospital beds and in rehabilitation centres. I tell them my story and always make it a point to show them my cars – sometimes even taking them for a ride. Often, that brief taste of freedom – the chance to experience the joy of mobility – is a transforming moment for them. I always look back on these visits with pleasure, especially if they end with a happy smile on a child's face. I believe this was the purpose of my disability – the message that I am meant to carry into the world. This is what makes me a . . .

## *Knight Of The Road*

I have covered long miles
With each trek giving birth to a new me
In wagons of different shapes and styles
Over the hills scanning horizons to see
Songs, bags and maps my load
Days, distance and destinations my code

A Sagittarius, I was born to run
From dusk till dawn I am on the move
Drifting with the shadows and the sun
Searching for myself, my journey – my love
Rising with the day and living through the night
As a knight I am inspired by stars bright

Each lane and line passed symbolises my glory
The humming engine is the power of my strength
Each mountain, valley and stream a line in my story
Every stretch of road a welcoming length
Just like weddings are walked up the aisles
My crusade is forever set on conquering the miles

I am a rebel with a cause
A rolling stone that gathers no moss
At times I set out just because
For one moment at a stand-still registers a loss
My home is the road and yes my grave
Come hell or high water – the miles I will brave

Lord knows I was born for the winding road
I am a *'Knight Of The Road'* . . .

# The Pencil Revolution

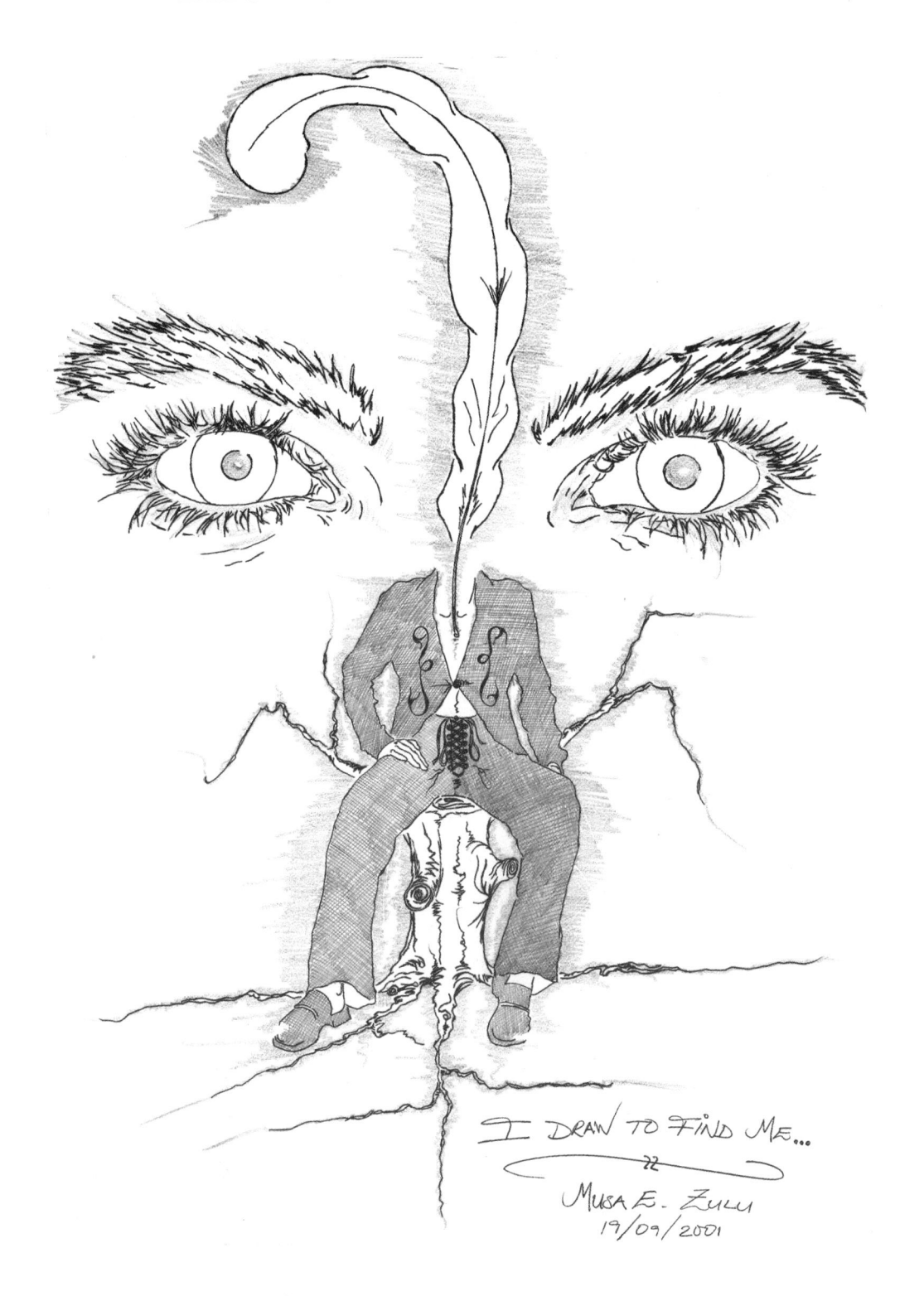

To me, drawing is more than a passion – it is what I do to find and define myself. It is a form of confession, a process whereby I express the truth about me and what is in my mind. When I draw, I create worlds and moments as I see and relate to them. I believe my drawings speak to people in different ways – they may convey messages that are boldly 'in your face' or play hide-and-seek, using more subtle symbolism. But whatever the strategy, all my sketches tell the same tale – the tale about me. My drawings do not only give the facts of the story, but the emotions associated with the events. Each sketch is a small world of mini-creation, fed from the streams of my subconscious. I have discovered that each time I draw, I reach down and touch the inner corners of my mind and soul, and that in the process, a part of me that I previously did not know about is uncovered and brought to life. As I walk through the miles of each of my drawings, I stir up a storm of images where the core of me is to be found. There is no other experience as exhilarating as coming to know myself through these creative storms and sharing my discoveries with the world. All the sketches in this book were drawn and framed to represent and freeze the particular moments, feelings and experiences I have gone through in my life. Some of them were done to put a 'visible' face to the poems and prose reflections I have written. Each has a special meaning to my soul.

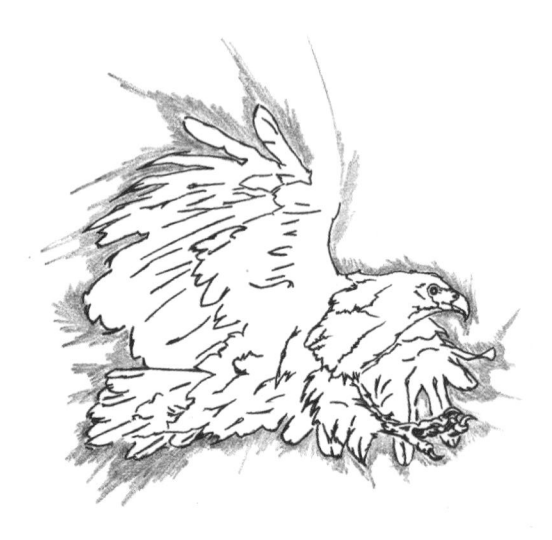

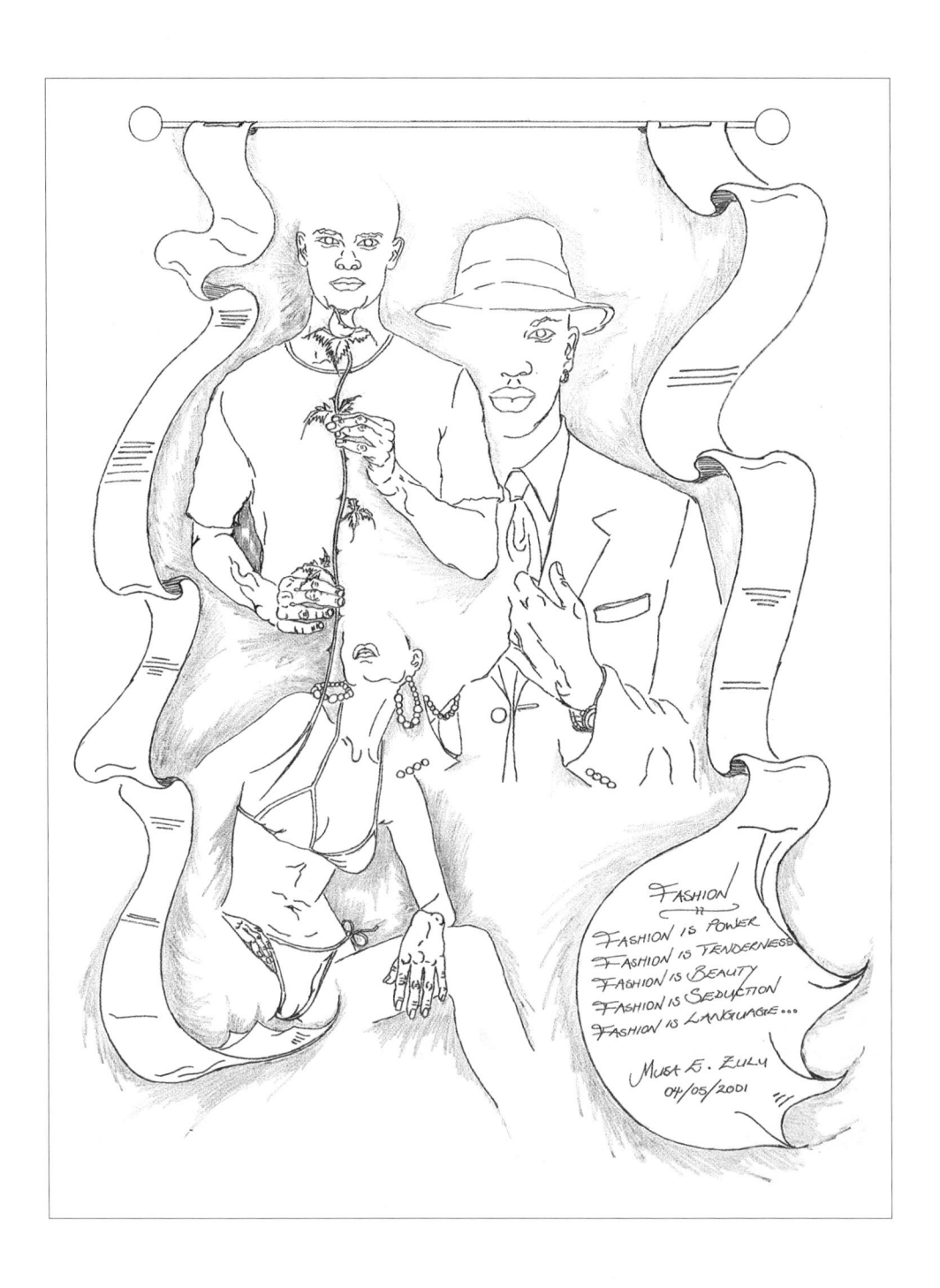

FASHION
"
FASHION IS POWER
FASHION IS TENDERNESS
FASHION IS BEAUTY
FASHION IS SEDUCTION
FASHION IS LANGUAGE...

Musa E. Zulu
04/05/2001

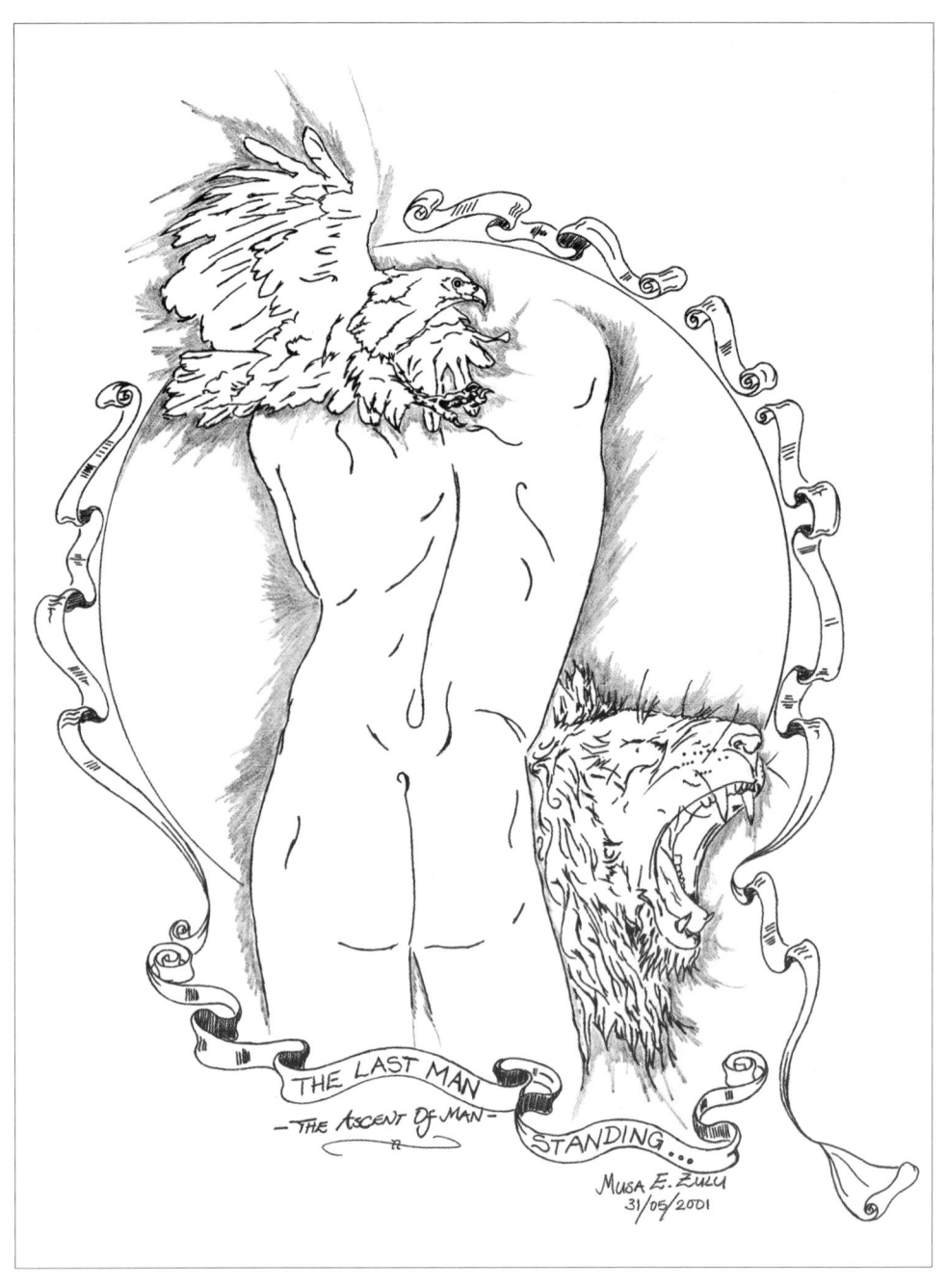

*He rules above the skies and over lands; he is the majesty of the towering mountains and the humble dance of the flowing rivers; he is the rays of light and the shadows in the dark, the flames of a fire and the frozen cold in the ice . . . The Last Man Standing . . .*

**M**any people have asked me why I choose to draw in pencil, rather than using colour and paint. My answer is that 'my hand married a pencil and not a brush'. I love my pencil style and I believe that if handled well, a pencil can create just as good a masterpiece as a paintbrush. It's what I refer to as 'The Pencil Revolution'. 'The Third World draws in pencil' – was my younger brother's joking response when someone commented about my refusal to switch to paint. The fact is that there was truth in his words; pencil is a very accessible tool and everyone can afford it. Our children in developing areas need to be encouraged to use their pencils to draw and not to wait for the brushes and paints that their parents and schools can't afford to make available to them. There is so much drawing talent out there that is lying dormant – and I believe there is no excuse for not activating it, because all it takes is a pencil to get everyone busy sketching.

I have also always believed that thoughts occur naturally against a background of black and white, where we are then at liberty to choose any colour and 'paint in' what we want to see and realise. Pencil offers me the opportunity to explore this philosophy and witness its reality and beauty. I love looking at my black and white sketches and projecting different colours onto them in my mind. I believe all of them are adaptable to any choice of colour and I love this flexibility that they provide – this is what I also find unique about pencil.

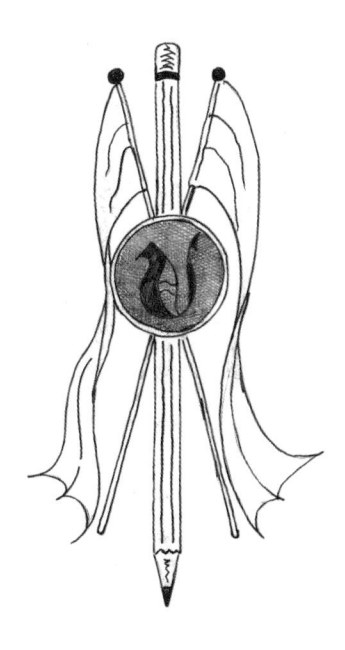

76

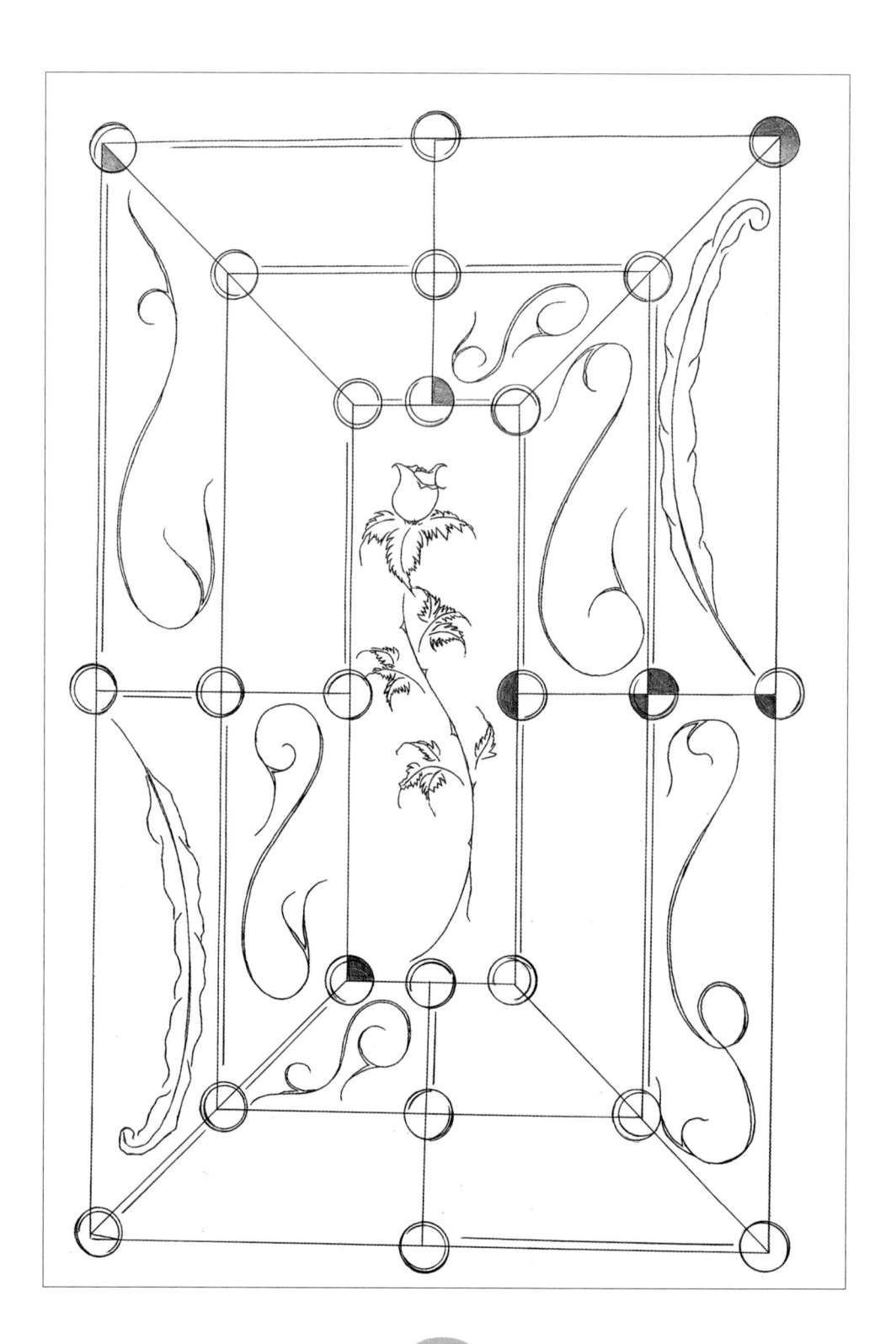

We all have our favourite symbols that hold special meaning for us – symbols that signify the relationships we hold with our souls, our dreams, our aspirations and views. I also have my chosen symbols, and they tend to recur again and again in my sketches. Many of my drawings have these features in common: a feather (at times dipped in an ink-pot), a rose, leaves, and swirling 'curtains', where I often write the titles of my sketches. These are my trademark symbols and each of them has been chosen for a reason. This is what they stand for:

### *The Feather*
*Wisdom:* I have always prayed and worked for this quality – for the wisdom to understand the depths of life and its mysteries. I dip my feathers in ink-pots to reflect on the art of writing and its power in shaping history, for I believe there is wisdom to be found in history and the lessons it teaches.

### *The Rose*
*Beauty Without End:* I consider it a positive attribute that 'beauty' characterises the relationship I have with my existence, my experiences and my surroundings. I have always looked on the beautiful side of life and I believe that if all of us were to adopt that outlook, there would be so much good that we could plough back into life – and so much richness to be gained from it. The powerful and universal symbolism of a rose will never fade with time. In the same vein, I want to live my life positively for as long as time allows me to be a part of this cosmos.

### *The Leaf*
*Growth and Diversity:* As a child of the diverse world, I have always tried to open myself to the wonderful complexity of life and nature. This is what the leaves on my sketches symbolise. I believe that the world has failed to note and sufficiently appreciate the power of diversity, and that if properly valued, diversity can lead to unity, not conflict. You may notice that in each sketch where leaves are featured, they rotate around and bind the drawing – this is my symbol for unity in diversity.

### *Swirling 'Curtains'*
*History and Time:* I am a product of history and a child of my times. Any soul who has no relationship with his or her history and no rootedness in time is, in my view, a 'floating' and hopeless soul. I want to belong, and I have found my sense of belonging in my understanding of my own evolution and my consciousness of where time has placed me today. This is what these swirling symbols signify.

"The Music Of My Scenes"

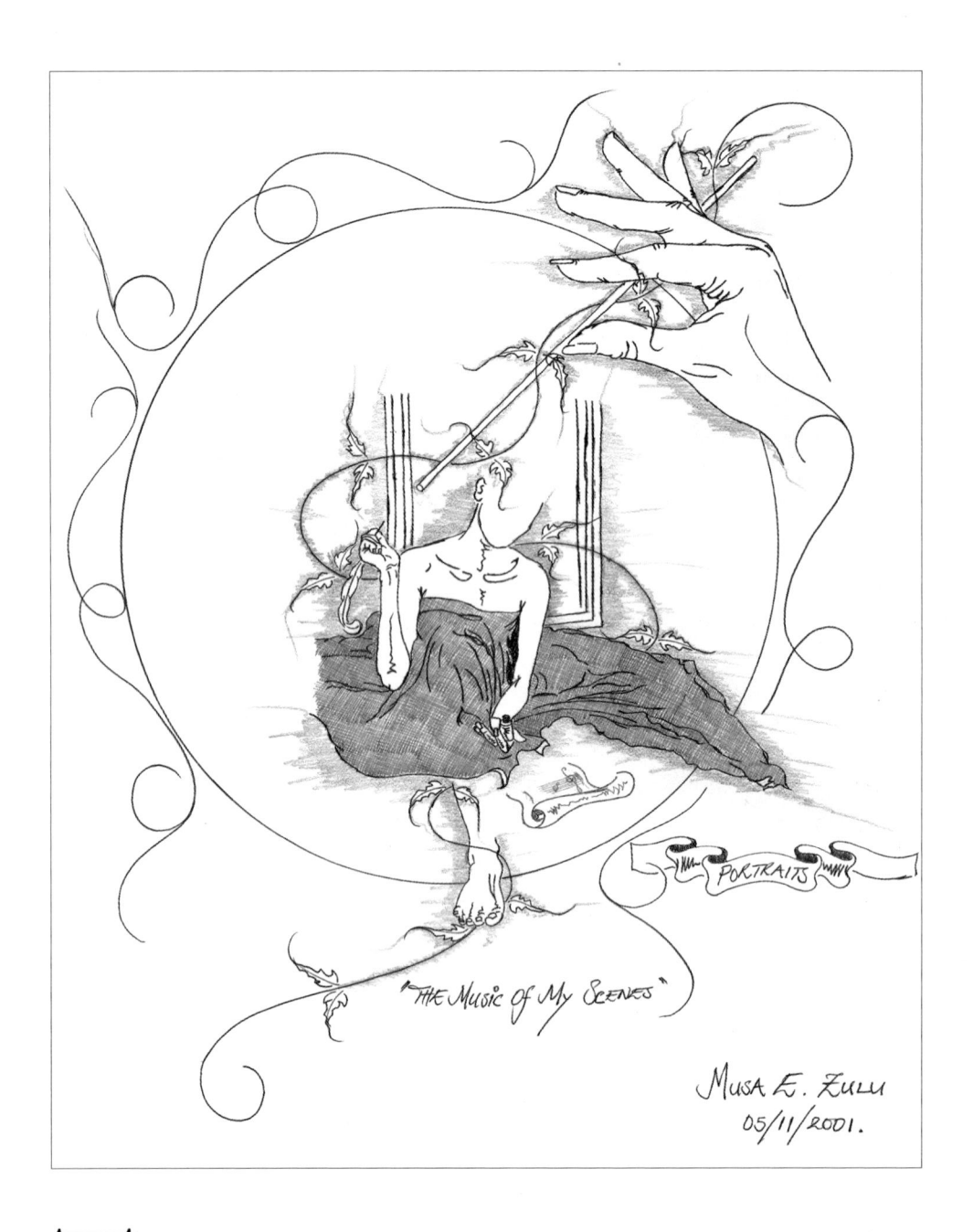

Musa E. Zulu
05/11/2001.

The world of thoughts, words, music and drawings is my natural element. This is where I find peace of mind and 'a quiet time' to communicate with my inner voices; the creative space is my home. I do not normally draw in the company of people, preferring to lock myself away, usually in my bedroom, where I sit on my own and listen to songs on the radio. I never feel alone at such times –

never lonely. I listen to the melodies and interact with the lines of the songs, the moods, instruments, musicians . . . producer. My mind becomes a traffic of thoughts that collide as they paint their pictures and silhouettes on the walls of my soul. When the songs reach their crescendo, I vault away in a cloud tinged by the spectrum of the rainbow which weaves its magical colours in the skies. I fly higher with the eagles and see the world from above, below and all sides. I swim deeper into the oceans with the whales in search of the fire and the flame, and explode to life with the whirlwinds and the storms. I am moved away from the immediate world of my fears and inhibitions – somehow in this realm, everything seems possible, beautiful and so true. This is where I find the silver-lining of life – the true vision of things. All that is left for me to do is to put it onto paper in a form that everyone can see and relate to. When the songs fade away and I turn off the lights, I go to sleep with a smile on my face and I dream in peace – because it is through these waves, storms and whirlwinds that my hand and the pencil have delivered to me another new drawing, that I will proudly exhibit to my brothers and the world the following morning.

I was still a young child when I discovered my love for drawing and the fact that I had the in-born talent to draw. My eyes were always attracted by pictures – those drawn by artists and those taken by camera. I loved paging through magazines and looking at the pictures of the world – through those pages, I felt like I was a traveller. But I was always most fascinated by the images that were drawn by hand. I found them amazing because they reflected another world – the world of thought. I wanted to make my own pictures and came to believe that this was the road I was born to walk – an artist's journey. One day I picked up a pencil and started copying and drawing the pictures I saw around me. I wanted to try my own hand at art – I longed to draw. Every skill is set to go through its trials and errors in order to grow, but in my attempts to draw I discovered that there was a natural relationship between my hand and the pencil – a duet that harmoniously sang its song to the beat of the picture scenes. I realised back then that I had the potential and ability to be an artist, and that if properly nurtured and developed, this was a talent that could take me far.

It took a while, however, for my own style to develop. In the beginning, I relied on 'copycat' sketches, drawings that I had copied from the various books and magazines that I read – all done in pencil. One of my heroes, an artist I still admire tremendously, was the legendary cartoonist, the late Jock Leyden. I was completely captivated by his imagination, skill and irony – by his amazing ability to marry art with humour in order to portray and provide biting commentary on the political and social issues of the time. His numerous cartoons spanned a broad range of topical issues, both local and international, and took me on a tour of the world, a journey of time as well as space. I took to copying his cartoons and was amazed at how closely my sketches managed to ape his originals; for a while, the cartoon became my genre.

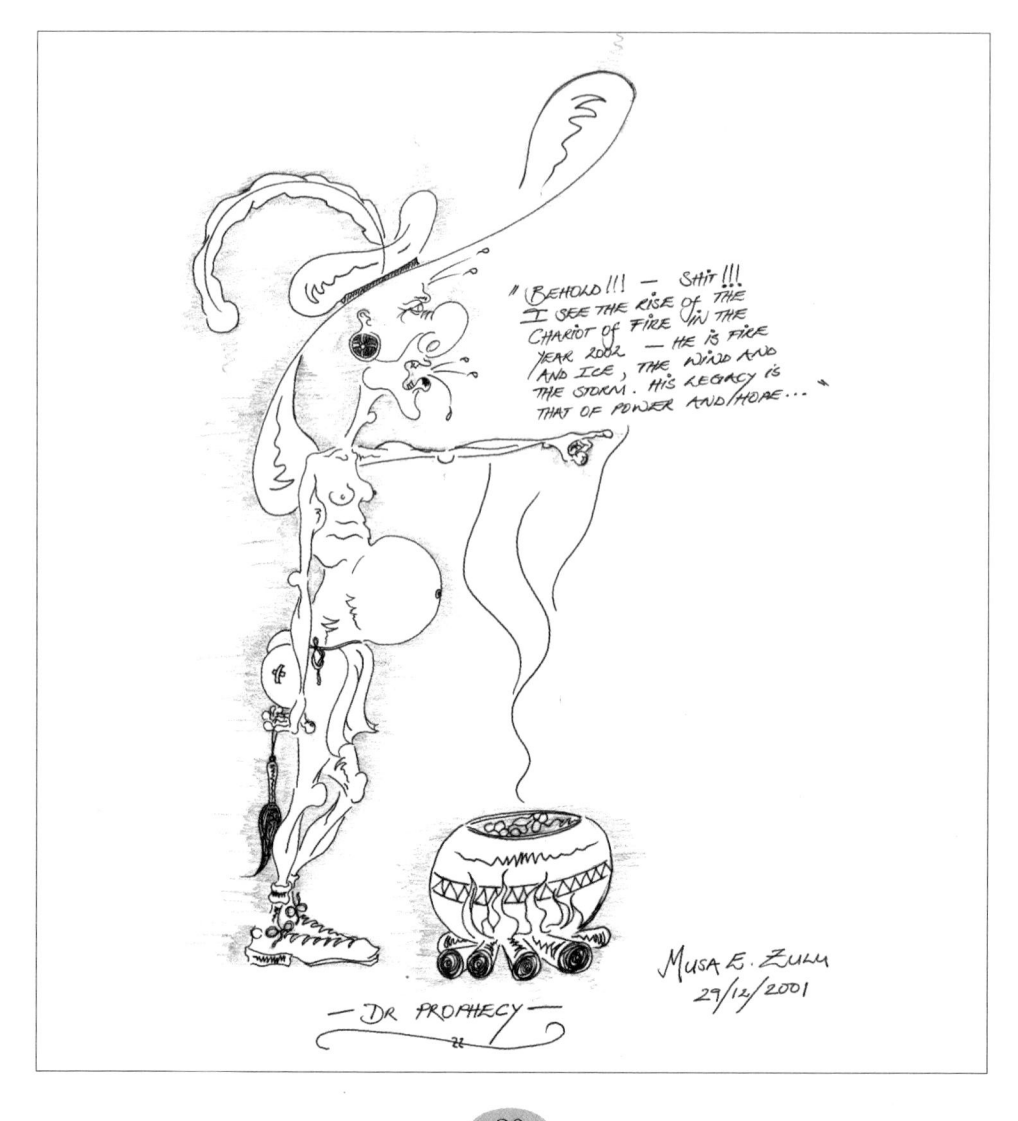

As time went on, I broadened my scope to more representational drawings, that depicted elements of our everyday lives – nature, buildings, vehicles, movie posters. I found I was an excellent copyist. At school, I didn't need the Biology textbook to be able to draw the heart, the body, the eye and other aspects of human anatomy. The hand and the pencil had imprinted these shapes on my mind through many repetitions.

This phase was an important one in my artistic development, refining my technique and honing my 'tools' to razor-sharp efficiency. However, I yearned to be not just a copyist, but an artist in my own right. My soul was crying out for expression, for its own identity through an individual style built on an independent spark of creation. I felt I had spent a lot of time as a copy-cat, living in someone else's shadow and viewing the world through other people's eyes. I always yearned to tell the story of life in my own way, through my own words and images, coloured with my dreams, experiences and perspectives. This yearning was partly what drove me to drop the pencil and abandon my hobby of drawing for a while. I needed time out to allow my psyche to catch up with my skill and to develop my own 'voice' on issues that affected myself and my world. Only then could I be an original and create drawings stamped with a style that only I could produce. In 1991, the pencil and my hand went their separate ways . . . It was to be nine years before 'something' triggered that hibernating relationship and brought the talent back to life again.

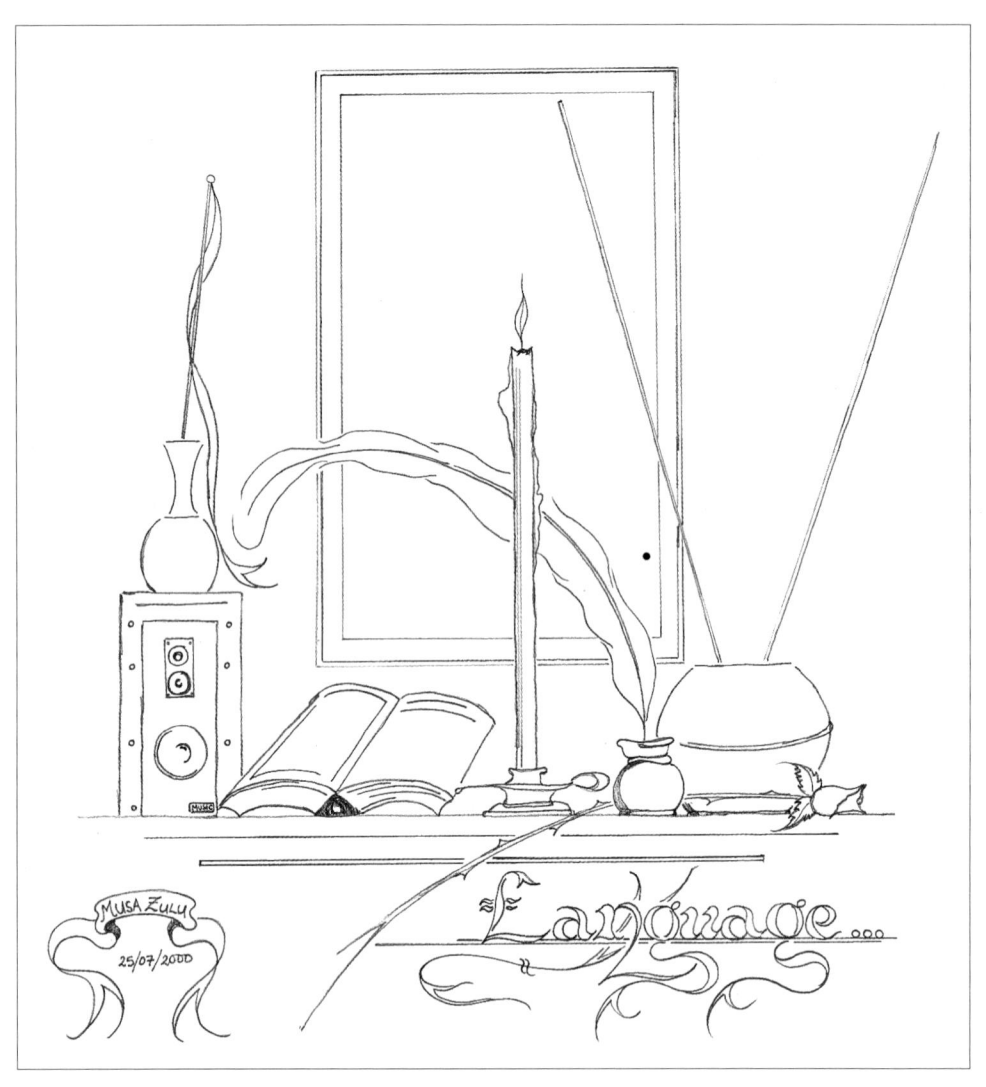

*Language is not only spoken words and thoughts expressed, but also the quiet of experience and perception. I love the word and I believe in its power. To me, language is everything, and everything has its own language.*

On a particular morning – the 25th of June 2000 – I woke up to find myself engulfed by the strong urge to draw. I climbed into my car and drove to town where I bought myself a big sketch pad, a set of good lead pencils, a rubber and a ruler – the tools of my trade. I went back to the house and with a smile on my face started sketching the story of my life and its various themes and relationships. 'Language' – my first sketch of this new phase – was born, and this time round the style was purely mine. I loved every moment of the two and a half hours it took me to complete the drawing, and I knew that I had finally found that vital inner spark of creation that I had yearned for. With pride I signed my name to it: 'Musa E. Zulu'. After that, there was no stopping the flood. The hand and the pencil continued to weave their magic in sketch after sketch until I had build up a pictorial collection of over 74 'portraits', each depicting a different phase, mood, or episode of my journey through disability and the various life changes and challenges it presented. Often, I found I was not just drawing the images of my mind's eye, but jotting down the thoughts that underpinned them . . . whispered lines of verse or prose that unconsciously guided my hand as it drove the pencil. It felt wonderful to be able to 'marry' the two great passions of my life under one frame and I often surprised myself with the final product.

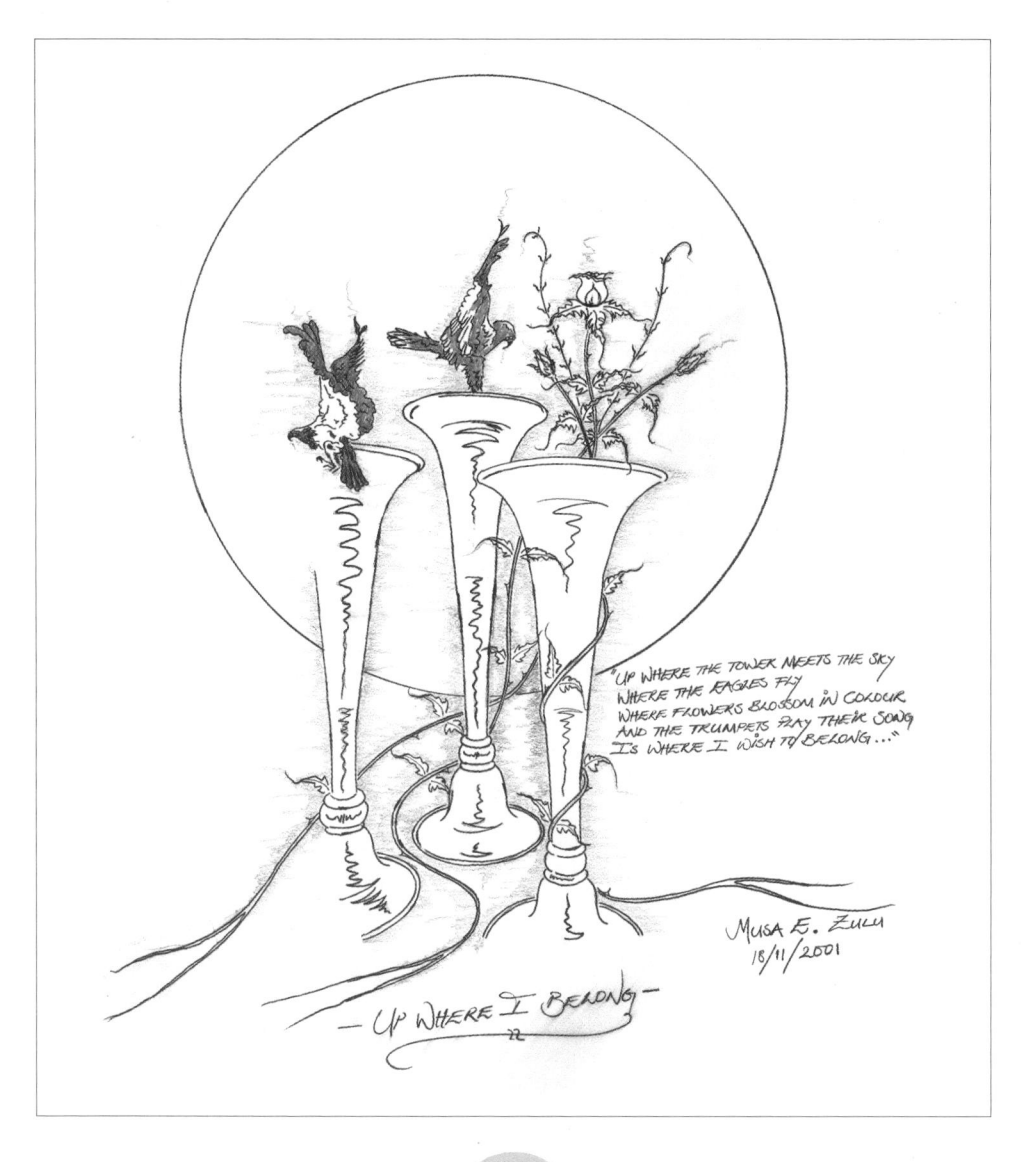

The collection of sketches displayed in this book represent the fruition of another dream. In 1995, when the car crash left me paralysed from the waist down, I resolved that I was going to continue with my life and hold on tight to what was important to me, never losing touch with my passions – particularly the passion of writing and drawing. I made myself a promise that I was going to use these two talents to document and give concrete reality to my 'adventure'. My sketches are the visual record of my life – 'the portraits of my thoughts' in the 'photo album' of my mind. If that album could be displayed in its entirety, it would have to be big enough to swallow the whole of life itself. It would need to be of gigantic size in order to do justice to the millions of pictures that go to making up the full story that is me. These invisible pictures are stored away in the private chambers of my mind as thoughts, memories and episodes of the many changes I have been through – these are my frozen times. Yet they are not solidified and fixed, but free-floating – and all I have to do each time I want to draw, is turn my eyes inwards and reach down into the infinite picture gallery for my inspiration.

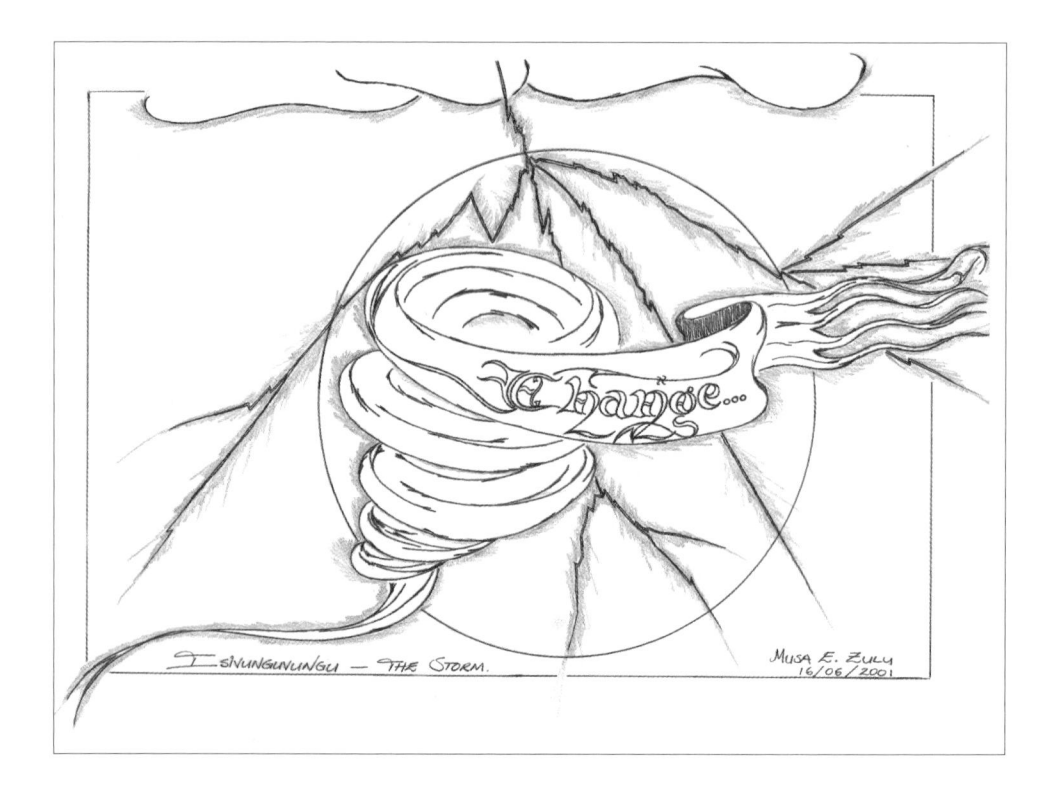

Isivungunvungu – The Storm.
Musa E. Zulu
16/06/2001

— Window of Hope —

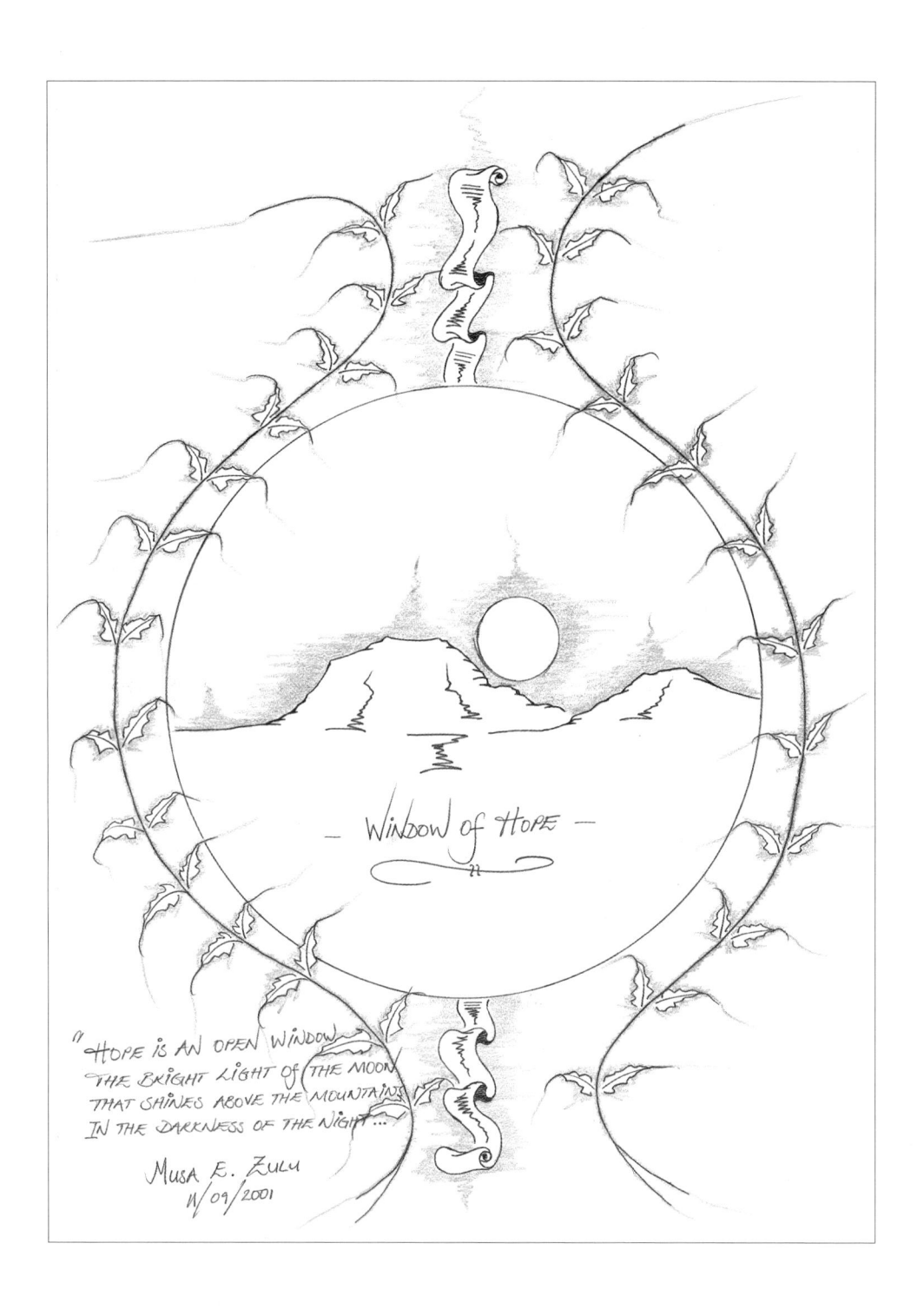

"Hope is an open window
the bright light of the moon
that shines above the mountains
in the darkness of the night..."

Musa E. Zulu
11/09/2001

**F**or me, life itself is a web of pictures, each of them expressing the beautiful language of creation. I write and draw to give face and sound to this language, using my pencil to 'paint' the pictures of life as I see and experience them. It is hard to explain to those who have not felt it, the wonderful feeling that is left in your heart after your talent comes to life and takes you to where you want to be – to who you really are. Always, when I finish a drawing I feel complete, fulfilled, defined and at home with both myself and the whole of life.

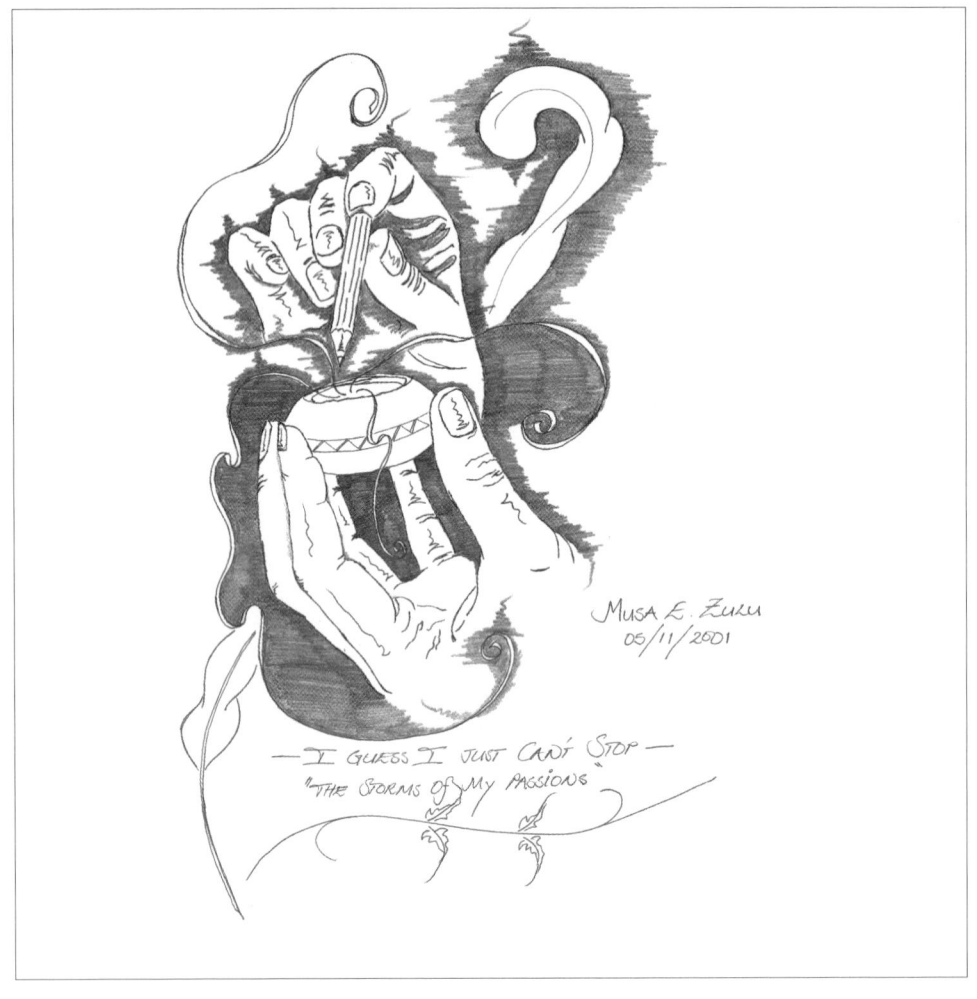

*I guess I just cannot stop, for every time I have completed one drawing or poem, and think I am ready to stop, another one unveils itself on the walls of my mind, its beauty and music tempting me to go on. I always accept this invitation to the dance floor of hand-and-pencil; I guess I just can't stop – these are the storms of my passions . . .*

# Scent Of A Woman

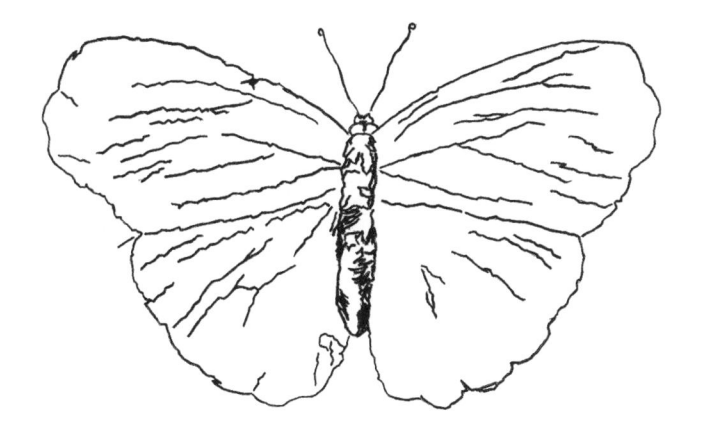

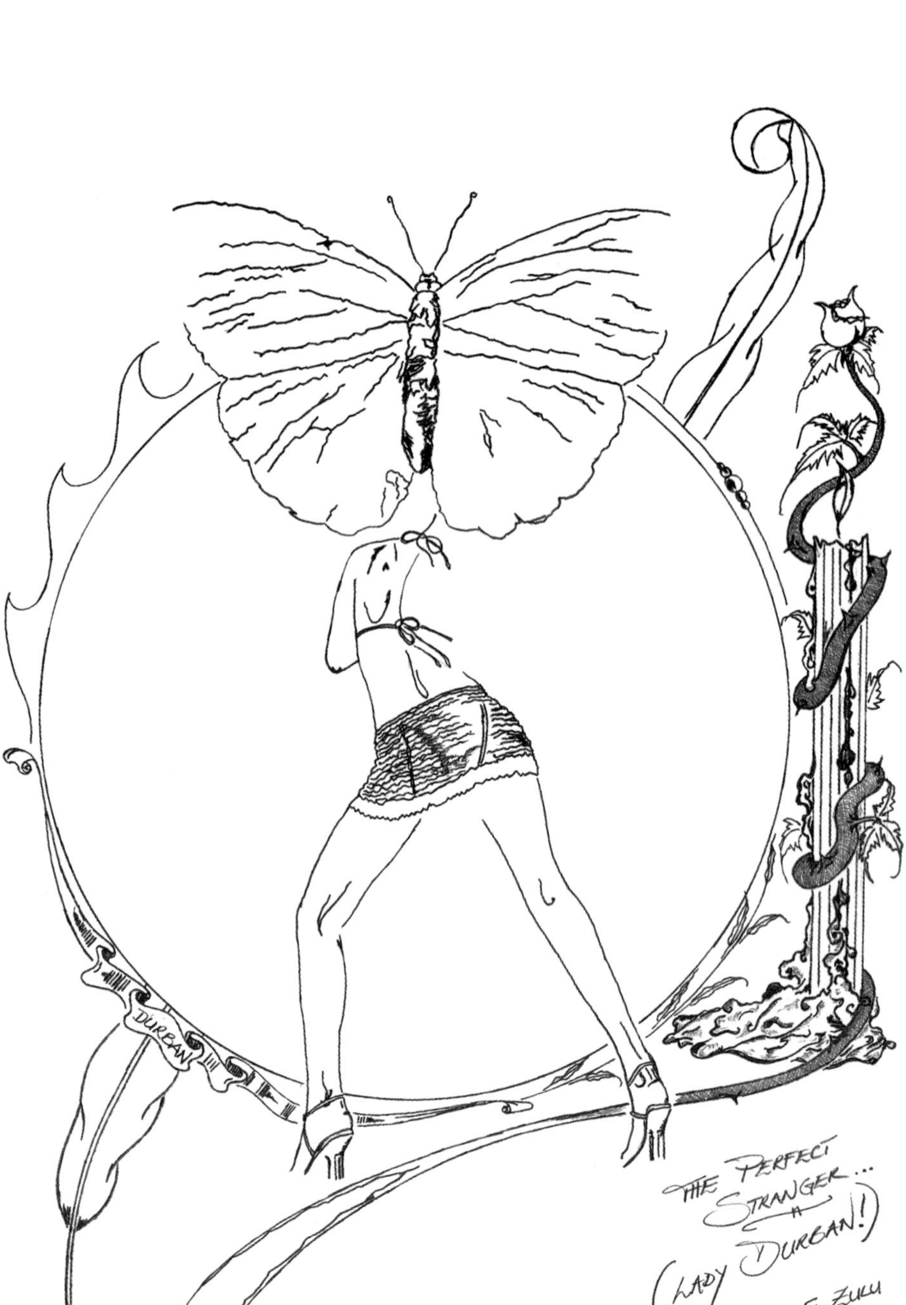
DURBAN
THE PERFECT STRANGER... " (LADY DURBAN!)
MUSA E. ZULU
07/05/2001

## *Perfect Stranger*

Winding down the busy West Lane
Of a city of a thousand footprints
Faces, new looks – strangers to the eye
Colours scattered by the touch of life
Sounds of a trader speaking his merchandise
Flags flying high with the commanding breeze
The sight of a porter, the posture of a gentleman
And the stranger at the corner

Standing there as if in waiting – is it for me?
Suddenly all life stands still, killing the wind
Like in a world where the quiet is too loud
The colour on the pole says 'pass' – they all do
But my eyes are locked on that pose of a goddess
For a moment I succumb to the power of fantasy
The scissors of Delilah weakening Samson

Stranger at the corner, beauty
You have stolen my breath away
Taken it on a wild dream to a world of visions
Where I had vowed I would never be caught
Tangling my soul in a spider web, prisons
Building entrapping walls all around me
Yet for now I want to be in these chains
And surrender all of my Kingdom's reigns

Like a shooting star she cuts through my skies
Moving forward like a siren on a catwalk
A short dress, sandals – the legs and the feet – butterfly
Flashing a stare that catches me from head to toe
Painting a smile that lights up the night, fire and candles
Making dreams come true without saying a word
'Quick, let me make a wish' – touch me, talk to me!
Tell me this moment has been worth waiting for

Stranger at the corner, give answers to these questions
Have you any idea what your spell has done to this man?
Do you know that the message in your song speaks to him?
Do you know that your stare is a gateway to his fantasies –
Your magic and touch, the key to the door of his prison
And your walk, his footsteps to freedom – tell me do you know . . .
That in the dock you stand accused, of love in the first degree?
You are guilty as charged, for Prisoner No.1 has now escaped . . .

I have always loved the company of women. 'I am the type of guy who gives the girl the eye – everybody knows', Paul Young sings in 'Wherever I lay my head . . .' Those words might have been written for me. To me, a woman is the music in the song of life, the poetry and the passion. I have always been intrigued by the power that women have in shaping a man's identity, personality and sense of self. I believe, as my grandfather always emphasised, that the pathway to the core of every man is through a woman. 'It takes a woman to unlock the full potential and liberate the true reality of what a man is and can be in his life,' he used to say. He always maintained he was of 'The Old School', and so am I. To be of The Old School means to be a practitioner of the 'gentlemanly' art of seduction; it is to understand that love is a game of skill in which the beloved has to be courted, not forced. I was brought up to believe that *'intombi iqonyiswa ngokweshelwa* – a woman is wooed and won by words.' The Old Man impressed on me that a man's language, if articulated well and creatively expressed, can paint the colours of his core and reveal the essence of the man in him.

Many people have questioned my 'over use' of women's bodies in my art; I have no apologies to give, only good reasons. The simple truth is that I love the bodies of women. To me, they are a symbol of natural beauty, perfection and sensuality – irrespective of their varying shapes and sizes. In my art, I use images of female bodies to reflect on the changing cycles of life, the intimate miracle of human existence embodied in the voluptuous sexuality of a woman's form. To me, sensuality is the essence of a woman, and this is why I love to draw her – to 'experience' her cycles of growth and feel the power of her beauty as she develops through the various stages of her life.

MASTERPIECE...

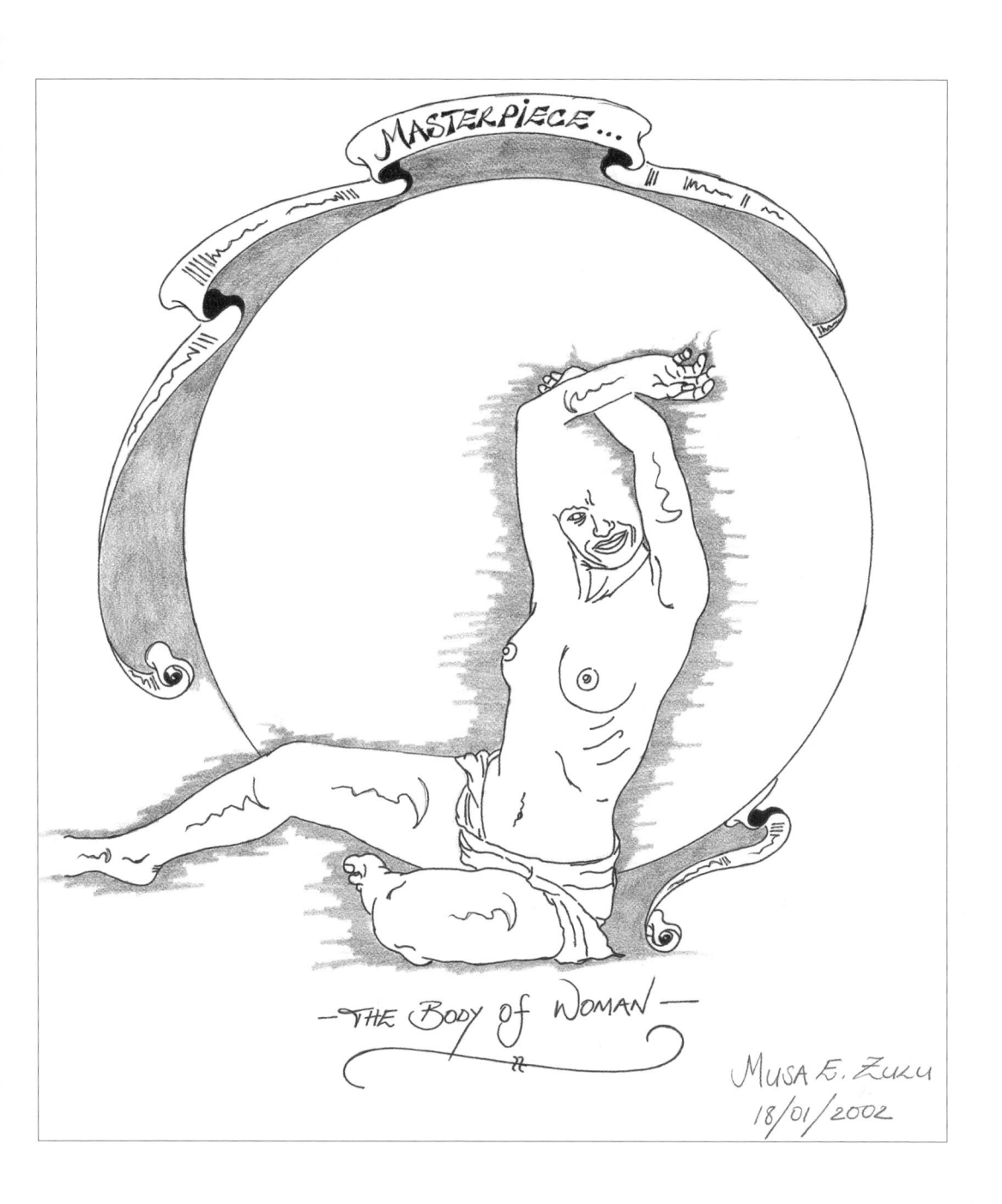

— THE BODY OF WOMAN —

Musa E. Zulu
18/01/2002

# *Unity And Love Without End . . .*

*My mother and I . . .*
*If one were to ask me one day*
*What of all lessons of wisdom I have learnt from this woman*
*I would proudly answer and say it for the world to learn*
*That she said*
*'Life is Unity, Beauty & Love Without End . . .'*

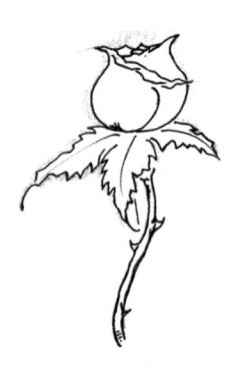

The sketch opposite is my mother's portrait. It features a blooming rose wrapped tightly around a burning candle – a collage of beauty that stands tall in front of a mirror, which in turn thrusts its reflections to the skies for the whole world to see, learn from and admire. I drew this sketch to reflect on the lessons of wisdom that my mother has taught me and the rest of my family. It is also the reflection of our bond and long-lasting sense of oneness in spirit and vision. My mother is everything I admire in a woman, the symbol of unity, beauty and love without end . . .

*Unity, Beauty, Love Without End...*

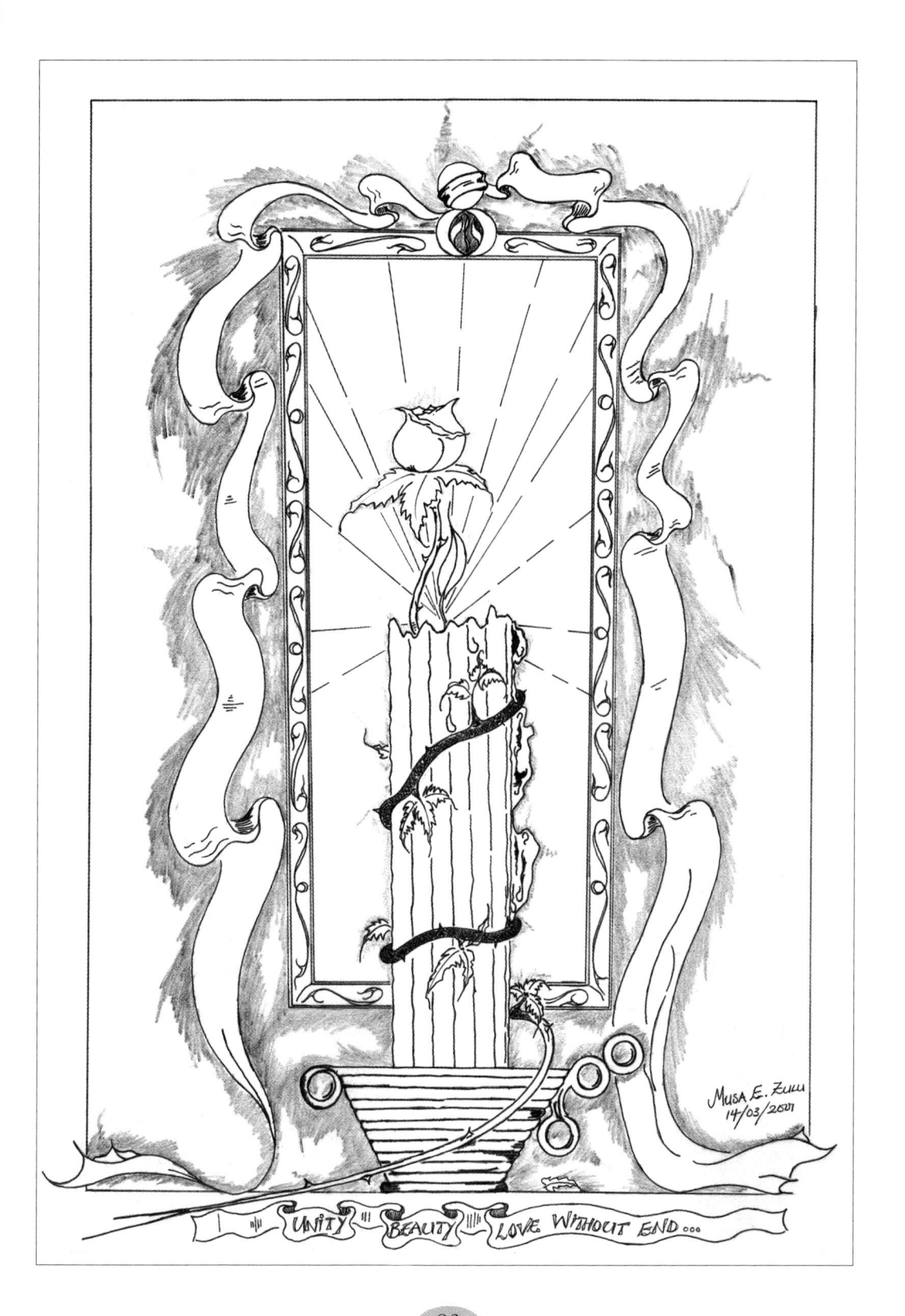

## *Let Me Be The One*

Let me be the One
The naughty story you whisper to a friend
That quiet dream that haunts your slumber
A stolen thought that triggers a smile
Your daydream, entombed in reflections
The sun and the stars, your man
Your confidante, let's kill the secrets

Let me be your song, your dance
Tell me lioness, where have you been?
Alone battered by the seasons, reaching out
Painting fantasies on grey walls and dark skies
A prisoner of despair, fear . . . searching
I ask you in my song, where were you?
Words whisper the painfulness of a love-hunt

Did he make you cry? I'll wipe away the tears
If he was not there for you, let me come closer
My ear is longing for your tale, if his was deaf
What kind of a man is blind to beauty?
A fool who only realises after the storm what has been lost
Let me carry you in a wave, give me a try
What kind of a man fails to cry?

Lady take it to the finish, hush!
Allow me to steal your fears away
Let my eyes marvel at creation, curves . . .
You are a sweet bite of tenderness, taste
That gently touches on a nerve, the pulse
I thought I had seen enough of this world
There is a universe inside your black eyes

Let me whisper to my friends about you and me
The nights and quickies, our naughty secrets
Fools will laugh and say I am crazy
If they ask me to go out, I want to be home
Waiting for the skies to clear and flowers to blossom
Let me shout to Heaven and Earth
For everyone who listens to know . . .

That you have Let Me Be
The One for you!

— THE GHOST
OF SEDUCTION —

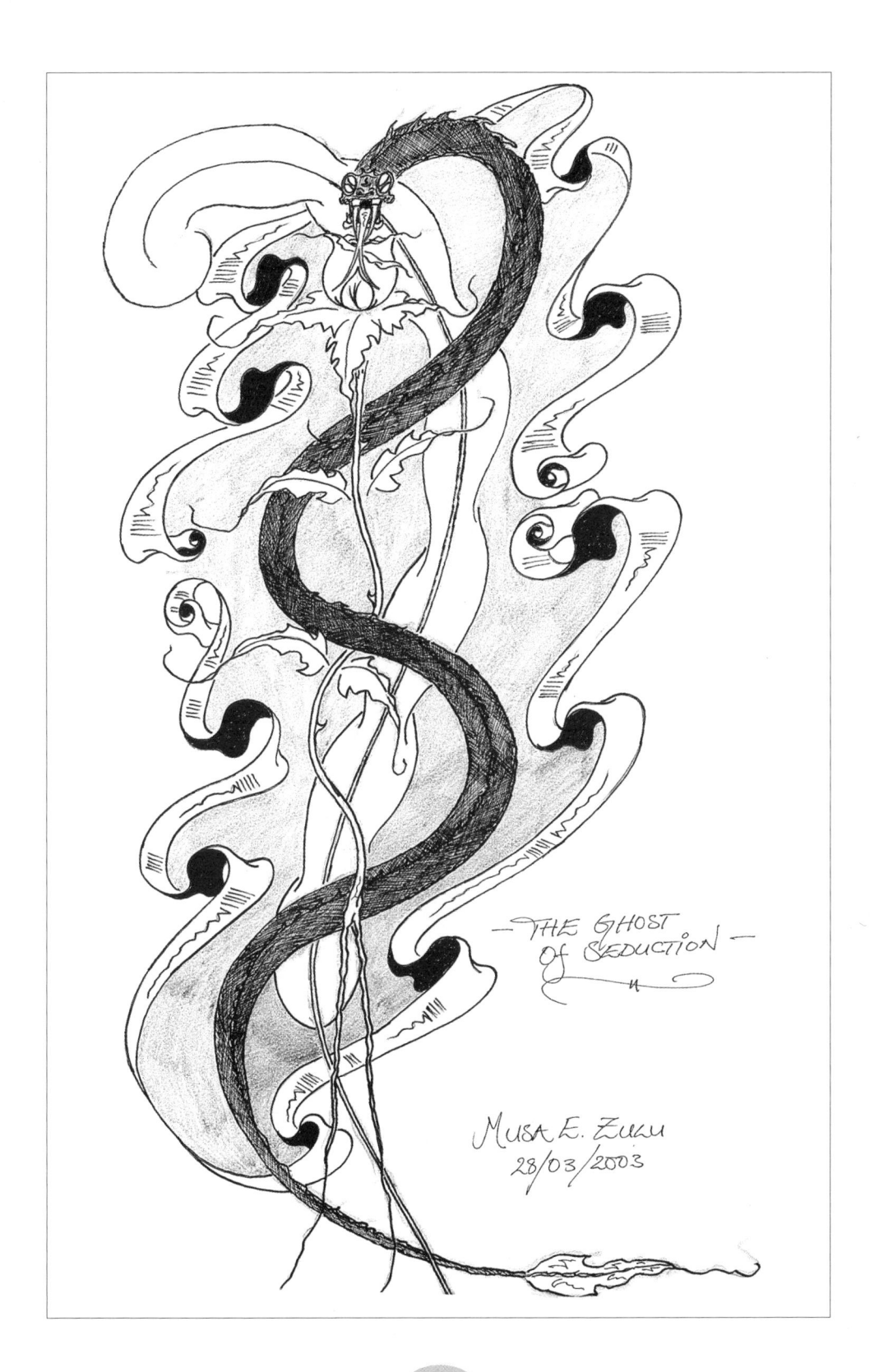

MUSA E. ZULU
28/03/2003

calculating not just his own moves but that of the other player. His goal is to know his woman better and find the spaces and places inside her soul where he can locate himself in order to light the fires of lasting passion that truly meet her needs.

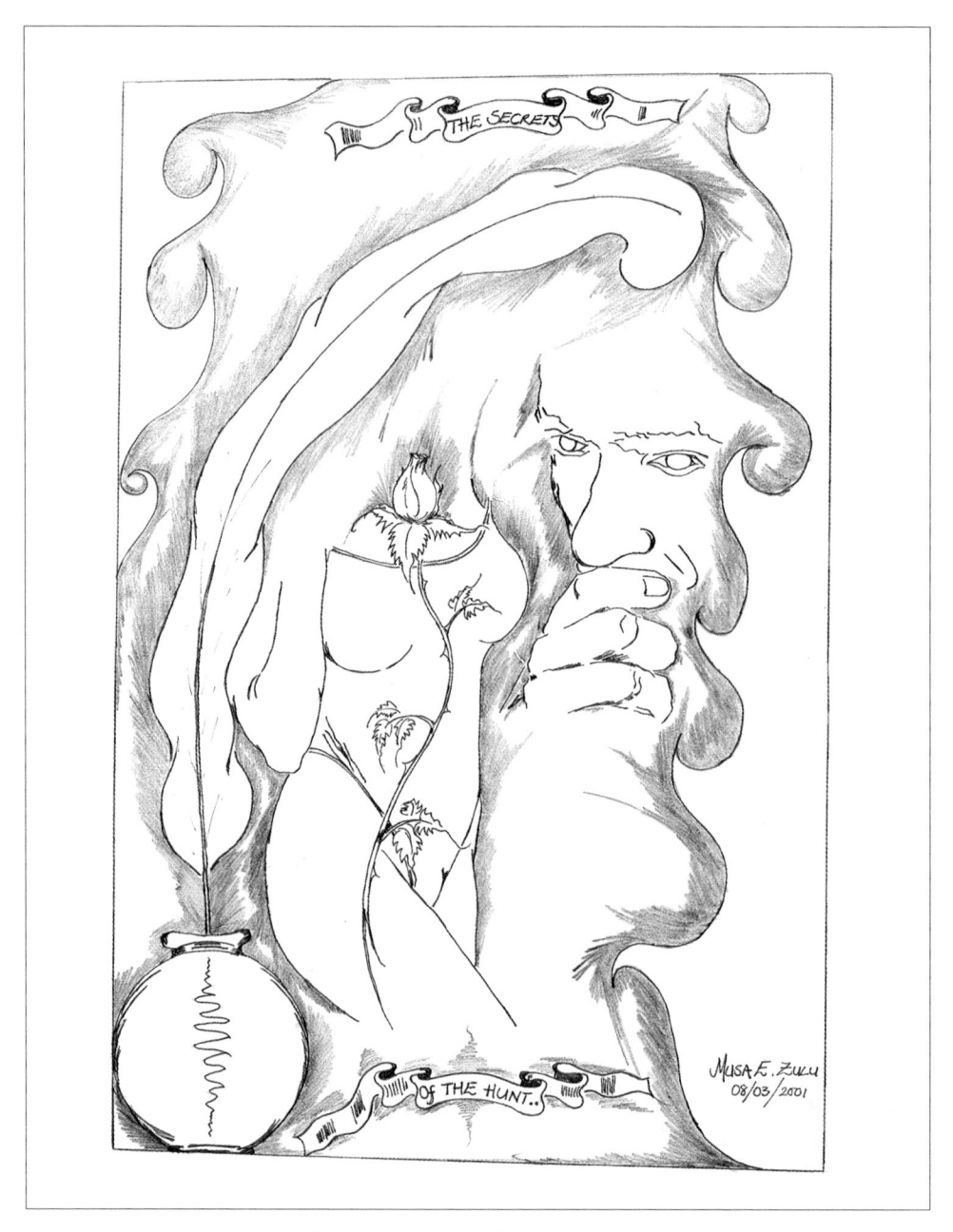

*The scent and the thorns of a rose*
*The untamed strength of the beast of desire*
*The surrender and the sacrifice*

Growing up in a township and interacting with other boys in the context of institutions, games and other forms of competition made me realise from an early age that part of ensuring a man's 'survival' in the masculine social jungle, and gaining the respect of the other boys, lay with the art of attracting women. Most boys dream of winning 'the best girl' at school and in the 'hood for himself, and I was no different. You could say that I was sexually aware from an early age. This was because most of my childhood was spent in the company of males far older than myself. When I was still in primary school, my uncles at home were sneaking off on their sexual adventures and staying out late. They would come back in the early hours of the morning to whisper and brag under the blankets about their 'naughty escapades'. At school, I interacted mostly with older boys from the standards above mine. I found this company much more stimulating than that of my own age-group – who spent most of their time chatting about weekend train rides to town and stealing into movie houses to watch karate movies without paying.

As teenagers, my friends and I used to sit and marvel at the older boys walking by hand-in-hand with their pretty girlfriends, at times kissing with closed eyes. We did all the adolescent boy things, drooling over the cover-page beauties in magazines, fantasising over the posters of supermodels on our bedroom walls. It was wonderful to dream about and yearn for that first kiss – the 'Day of Confirmation'. I loved watching movies about lovers on TV and paid special attention to the language and the music that was used to shape and transmit the message of love. What I saw and heard I then replayed in my own way to secure my own victories.

The sketch on the opposite page sums up my approach to romantic encounters, giving form to the dual desires to experience the full sensual pleasures of love while finding a more permanent home in its embrace. I was taught to respect a woman and never to push things too far with her unless I was sure that she was willing to play along. So this sketch speaks of my belief that love in its truest form is a democracy of the soul, and that its constitution upholds the principle of respect. The woman in the sketch has no face – the rose is the core of her identity. The rose represents inner beauty, desire that cuts across the physical body to display its true colours in the home of the soul. The man is captured in a pose of reflection – the poker player pondering 'the secrets of the game',

**M**y first break with relationships came when I was in Standard Six at Ogwini Comprehensive High School in Umlazi, Durban. I was just thirteen years old and knew very little about the world of women, except what I had heard from the many stories that the older boys told to us. 'She' was tall and pretty, young and playful. I must confess that to this day I do not know what I said or did to win her hand. I was still young and gathering my experiences – we were both learning the ways of love.

Fourteen years later, after a string of relationships and encounters (both failed and successful), I sat down to reflect on the art of courting and 'going out'. These reflections gave birth to the poem opposite, which – had I had the skill to write at the age of thirteen – I would have loved to have presented to my first love . . .

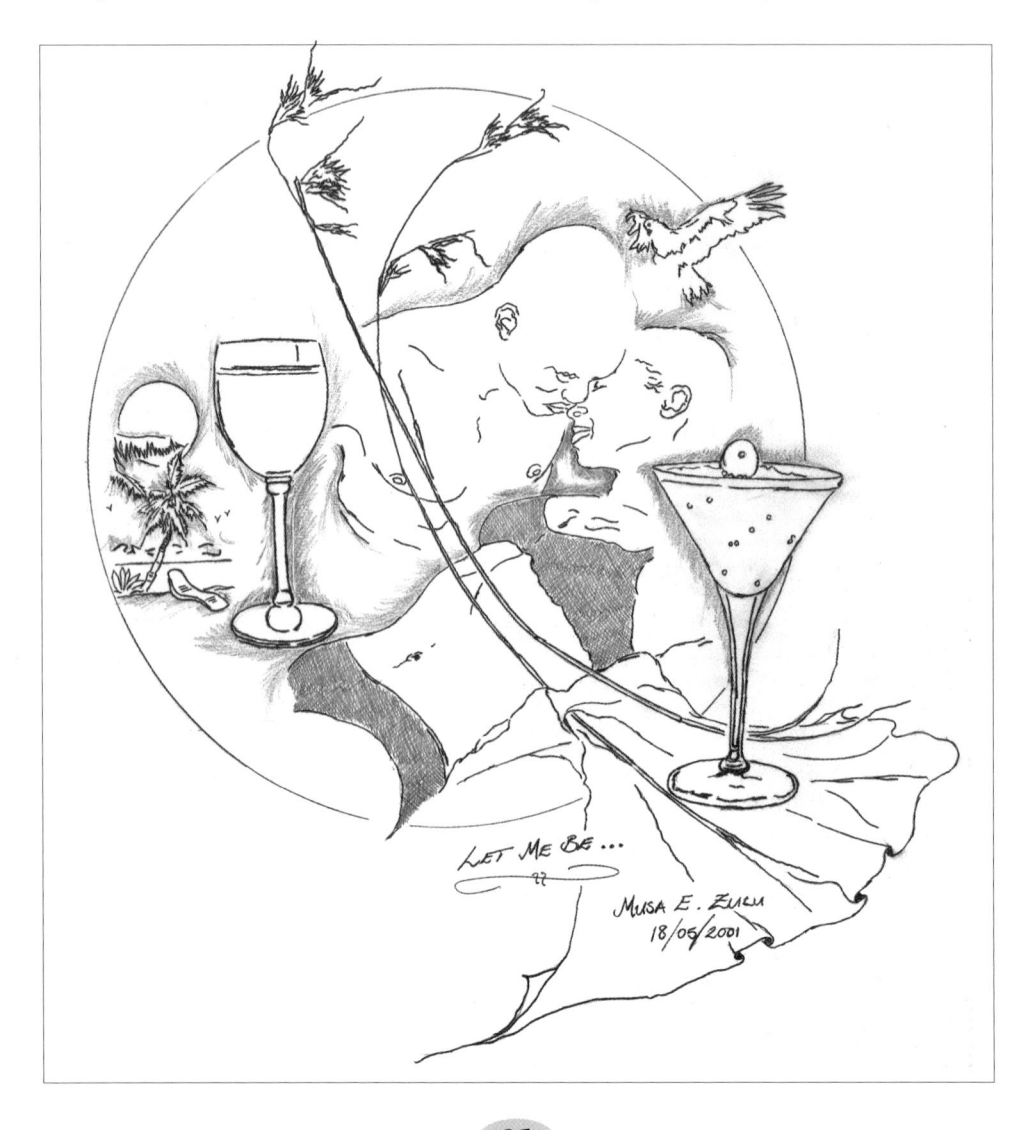

## *The Ghost Of Seduction*

Come on, I'm waiting
Enslaved in raw fantasies
Tortured by wild dreams
Come on, I'm here
Arms and mind opened wide
Deliver me to the war of passion

Wrap your arms around me
Break me like a python
Eyes of a cobra in deadly anticipation
Poison me with your gentle bite
Touch me, feel me, taste me
Drug me in eternal seduction

Sweet lips soft as petals
Sharp nails, the thorns of a rose
Hungry fingers, tear me apart
Explode like a fire
Freeze me like ice
Surrender, give in to me
Roll your tongue on my horn
Yours is mine, don't you mourn
Take me in, baby open up
Every man's wealth, the pot of gold
I want to be there
Back and forth is the direction I'll take

Grab me closer to your silky skin
Smear me with oils and perfume
Bathe me in your violent embrace
Lock me inside your prison
Whip me with the sting of your scorpion's tail
Be the master and I'll be your slave

Open your eyes, let me read you
What are your dreams, what do you feel?
Part your lips sending a soft message
'I'm coming' did you say?
Wait for me, for where you go I want to come
Let's take this journey together

The sketch on the previous page and the poem that accompanies it offers a 'male's eye view' of desire. It epitomises male surrender to the power of passion and the 'quiet command' that women can exert over men through the mastery of seduction. In this case, the traditional roles of male control and female subordination are reversed; the man is in the begging position, the woman the dispenser of favours. The sketch and poem evoke the two extremes – wild and tender – that for me make up what I refer to as the 'paradox of love', that is, love as 'liberated enslavement', and love as a feeling of 'gentle force'. They convey my preoccupation with the erotic power of women, my belief that love is a free relationship conducted by two willing partners, and that the core of a man is expressed not through his brute strength, but through his tender and creative side.

I have spent a lot of my life chasing love. Like many men, I often confused love with the erotic thrill of the hunt, the 'gentle kill' that celebrates 'the untamed strength of the beast of desire', the endless quest for the transient pleasures of the flesh. True love changes all of that; it humbles you, softens the macho ego. Love stops being the trophy of the perpetual hunt and becomes the liberating exchange of true intimacy.

When I met my wife Jay-Jay, I knew instantly that she was 'the one'. I first saw her on a crowded street, walking past my car, and her beauty leapt out at me. I commented to my brothers right there and then that she was 'born to be my wife'. I rolled down my window to speak to her; she said 'Hi', and I said – 'I love you!' That might sound crazy or presumptuous now, but I was only obeying my mother; she had always told me I should confess and surrender to my love if it was genuine. Jay-Jay gave me her number and that evening I phoned her. We spent the whole night talking and exchanging SMSs. I didn't tell her I was in a wheelchair. This was very unusual for me, since I always made it a point to declare my disabled condition to the women I met. But with Jay-Jay, I just couldn't do it. I was too terrified that she might exercise her discretion and walk away. The next day we met for a date, and I still didn't tell her. She climbed into the car and we rode about and talked, and I read her one of my poems, 'A Quiet Time'. It was the first time I had ever read a poem of mine to a woman. It struck me later that in all those early encounters, I spoke to her in English, not Zulu. I was so blown away by her beauty that she forced me into another language! To me, it was no surprise to learn that she was from Swaziland. I have always been a wanderer by nature, and in Zulu we have a saying: '*Induku enhle igawulwa ezisweni*' – roughly translated it means 'A beautiful stick you will find in places far away'. When I finally did dare to mention my disability to Jay-Jay, her comment was: 'Oh, so this is why you drive with your hands.' She had already figured out what there was to know for herself. All I could do was laugh sheepishly and relate my story to her, hurrying to assure her that I was now back in full control of things. A year later, I proposed and was elated when she agreed to be my wife. We were married on the 25th of January 2003. The sketch below expresses the love I feel for her.

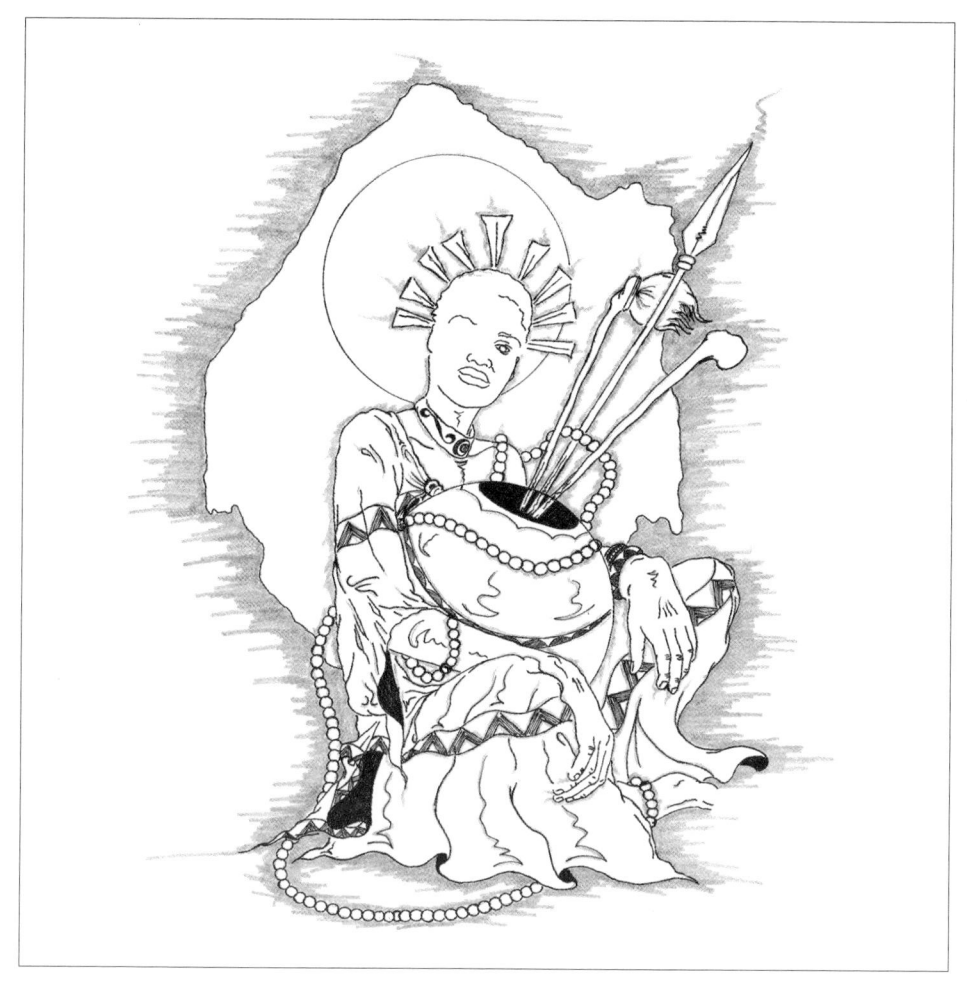

***For Jay-Jay***
*Love to me is the poetry of sharing*
*A tale told in a lover's prayer*
*So touch me and whisper to me*
*Your language of Love*
*For Love to me is You . . .*

# A Different Corner

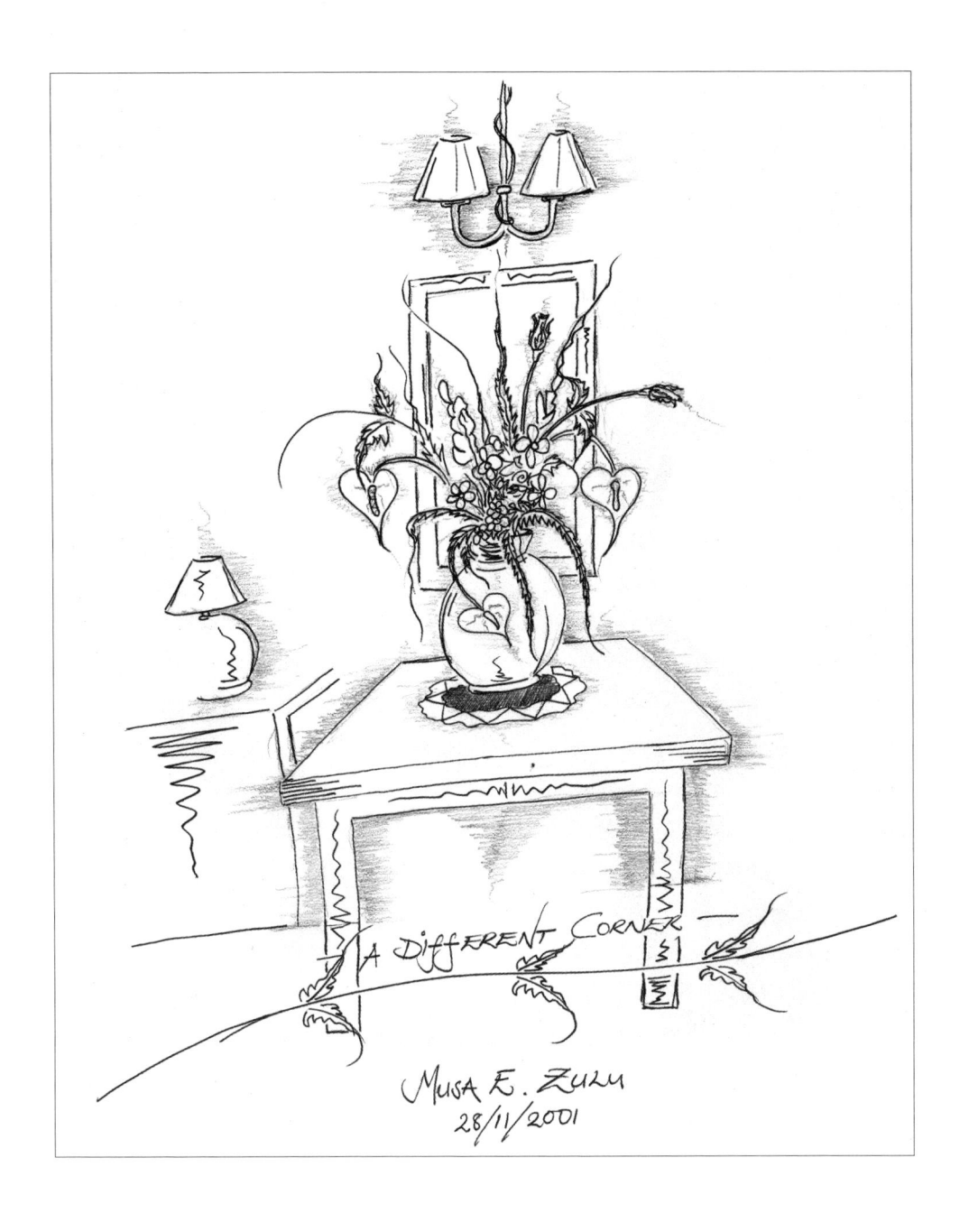

# *A Different Corner*

There is so much you could learn
So much you would understand
About the world of the other on the other side of the fence
If today you made a commitment to a new path
That takes you away from here to a different corner . . .

You would come to know how they live their lives
– what they understand . . .
And what they cannot understand about society and its order
The world is big and its oceans and rivers are wide
A lot of what happened with time has left its aftermath
You will not find it here until you have seen a different corner . . .

There is no need for high walls for they cannot stop the storm
– it was the waves of change that brought us here my friend
It is an explorer who comes to write tales about life and its borderlines
The different faces and places, the colours and the shades – history and the blood-bath
All of this you will find painted in the shadows of a different corner . . .

We were all taught to use the same path when we go home
– reasons were given as to why this and not the other one . . .
And we have been taking the same route to our schools and fields ever since
But life is a convolution of pathways that connect somewhere down the line
This is where we ought to share the experience of life, not from the comfort of our familiar stand
Life is about this principle; so let's take it with us to a different corner!

**N**one of us is born as an island. We are all children of a society, and every society has its different and diverse cultures. I have always wanted to be an integral part of this diversity. Growing up in South Africa has made me especially conscious of the need to change our attitudes to 'the other' – to experience the similarities as well as the differences between us, to bridge the divisions that set us against each other and find one another in our shared humanity. I don't believe that one automatically qualifies as a child of The Rainbow Nation simply by virtue of having been born into it; you earn your place in its ranks by going out and touching the rainbow – allowing yourself to be washed in the colours and be a part of, not apart from, the spectrum.

Yet it takes courage to emerge from the comfort zone – the cocoon of your given unit – into the wider world, where the storms of controversy hover, where 'the other' does not know you and you do not know them. This is even more true for a disabled person. It is tempting to remain in your familiar corner. But it is in the outer world where life in the full sense of the word is to be found, and this is where the relationships that make up the complete face of life are also to be found. No matter what our circumstances, we are all called on to go out into the world and be a part of its developments. This is where we will meet the other in equal exchange, mingle our 'colours' into new and unique combinations, and experience the full beauty of life's harmonious diversity that makes it possible for the rainbow to shine in all its glory . . .

**A**ll rivers end in the ocean, but each carves its own unique route to its destination. As much as I celebrate the equality and oneness of our common humanity, I also believe it is important to hold onto the identity that gives us our unique difference. As a child of the universal rainbow, part of what gives me my 'colour' is my ethnic character. I grew up in a KwaZulu-Natal township and had strong ties with my grandparents' rural households – these are the worlds I can say I truly know.

I am a proud descendant of the house of Zulu, and I have never been happy with the stereotypical image that has come to be accorded to my people – 'aggressive', 'war-mongers', 'uncultured', and the like. In the poem and sketch that follow, I have made a deliberate attempt to distance 'the Zulu' from all the usual clichéd associations – the animal skins, drums, shields and spears – taking him away from his history as told by someone else and depicting him from my own perspective. For I believe that it is when someone else tells my story that the stereotypes intrude. I wanted to depict the beauty, wisdom and maturity of my culture, and for that reason

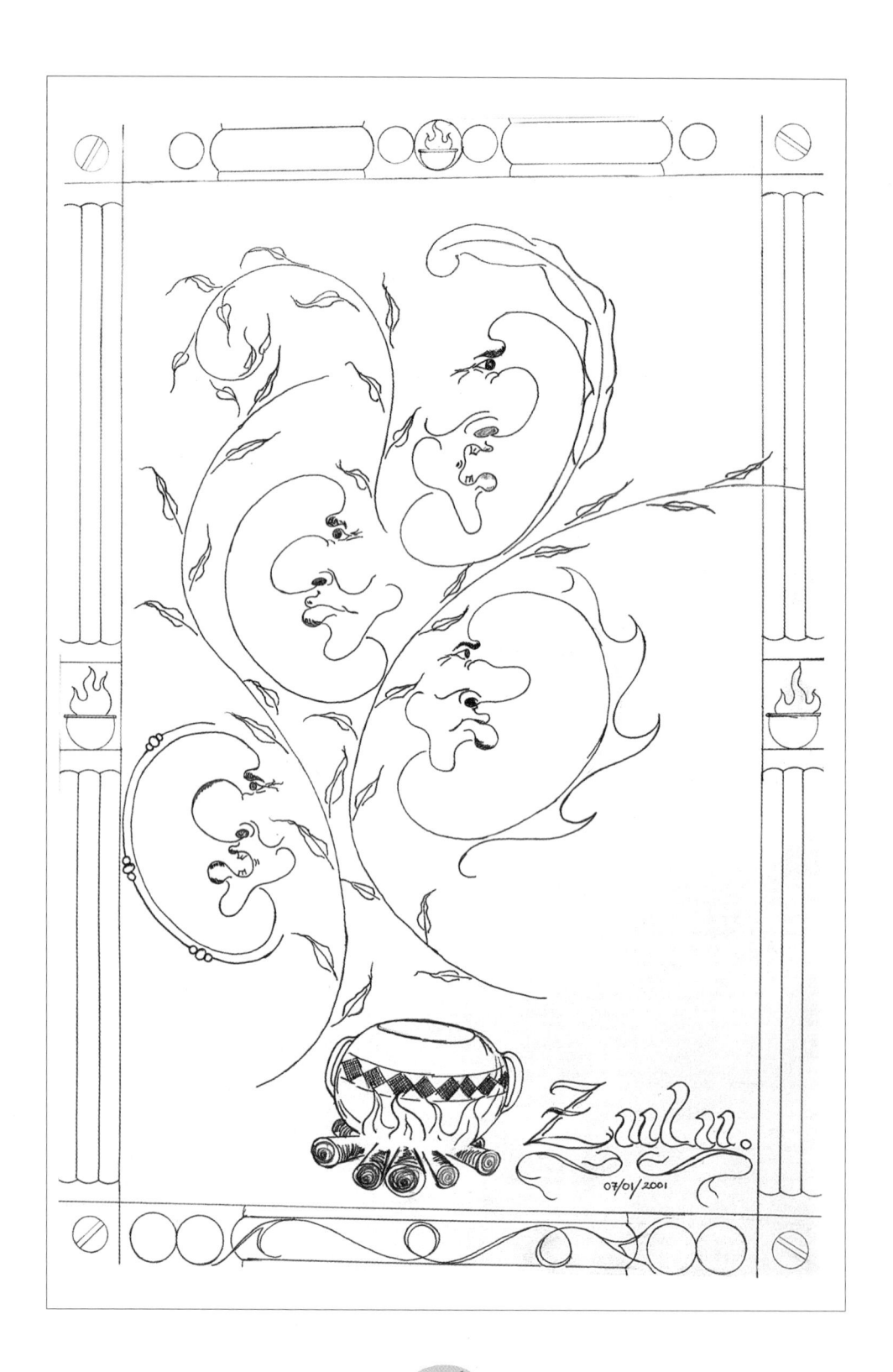

I chose images of talking and listening heads, of sharing and continuity. History teaches us that the house of Zulu was a lineage of warriors who went out and conquered others in order to expand themselves into a nation. For many, this might sound like colonialism, but to me this movement represents 'the art of continuity through the tides of destruction'. This majestic crusade of the Zulu people aimed 'to plant a tree that feeds generations in unity'. It was a process that unified diverse cultures and mobilised them around a common objective of nationality, peace and togetherness. The 'trees' that weave through the drawing symbolise this growth and continuity, with the adjoining leaves depicting common origins and an appreciation of diversity. The feather positioned above all the other symbols inside the sketch reflects the wisdom of a people. For a Zulu, the ultimate revelation of wisdom lies in the art of seeing no difference, in appreciation for the traces of diversity among those of a common ancestor. This, to a Zulu, is the true essence of family. The calabash on the fire depicts the tradition of sharing and warm relations that contribute to amicable interaction. The bolted pillars on the edges of the sketch point to the strength of common purpose that derives from unity, while the fires that burn everywhere signify the past, present and future of a people guided by light.

# *Zulu*

A Zulu is not only about the pounding drums and dance
A Zulu cannot only be defined by his spear and shield
Nor does his courage on the battlefield portray his whole nature

A Zulu talks and a Zulu listens
His silence is his peace and his voice his command
His eyes are always focused on building his world
And in them burns the spark of his inner strength
The wrinkles on his face mark his determination
To plant a tree that feeds generations in unity

This is the secret of his wisdom
His master plan revolves around family
A Zulu shares his soul with those around him
This is the wood that fuels his fires
The winds of change only see his flame burning higher
For his sense of togetherness is the bolts of his culture

His history is about survival
The art of continuity through the tides of destruction
His legend tells of a mystery of diversity in unity . . .
Oneness

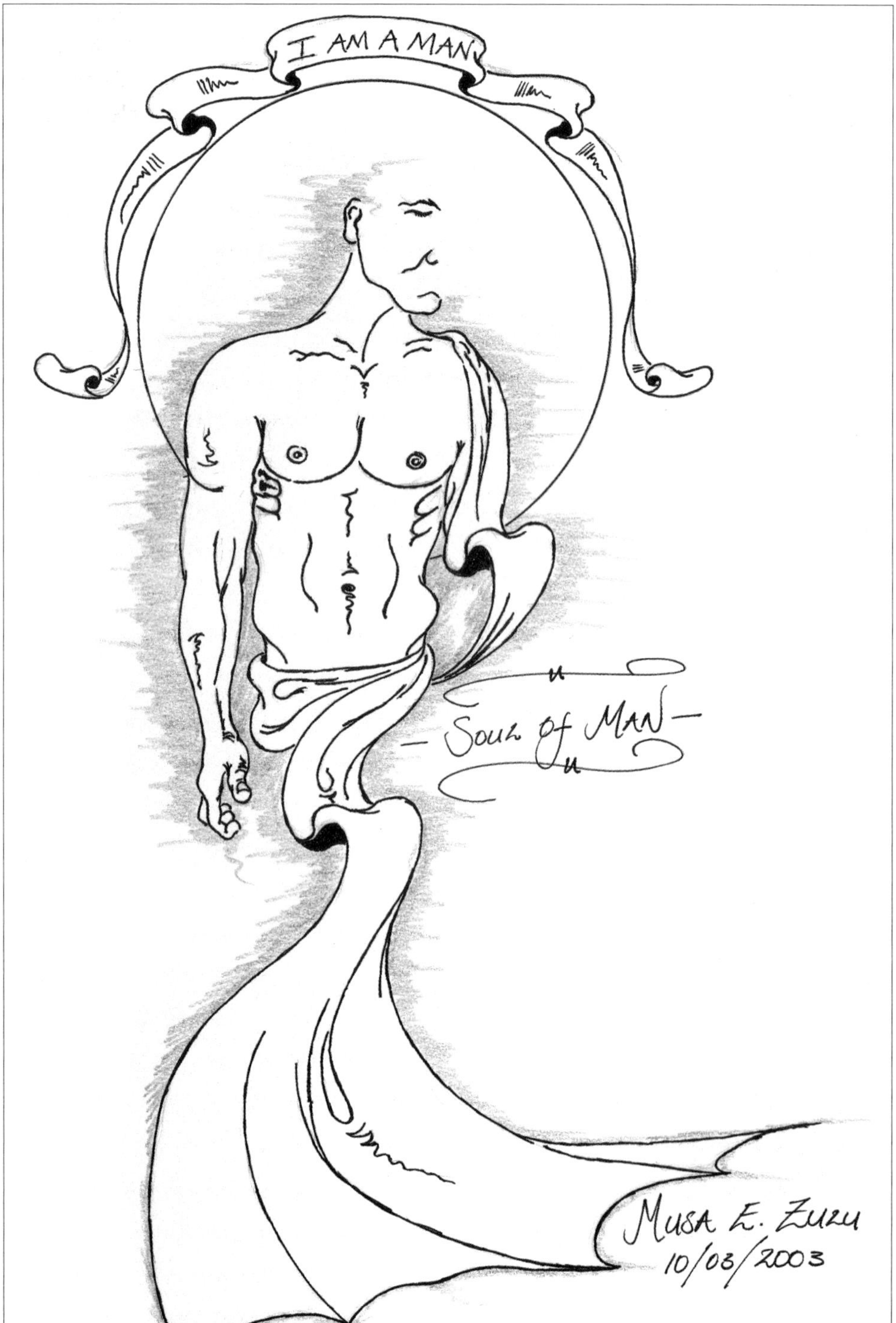
I AM A MAN
Soul of MAN
MUSA E. ZULU
10/08/2003

It is not always easy to be a man in this life, especially coming from a culture like mine, where so many expectations are placed on men. It is even more difficult to be a 'different' man in a society conditioned into negative attitudes and stereotypes about shades of difference. It is hard to lift your head high and stand tall in a world where the weight of discrimination sits on your shoulders. Disability is one of those shades of difference that is discriminated against in our society. Stereotypes strip disabled people of their dignity, their sense of control over their destinies and their ability to express their potential, their dreams and desires. This is why so many disabled men find it so difficult to establish relationships with women – society alienates them from their manhood, since it defines them as being less of men. As with so many things in life, the road to social acceptance has to start with self-acceptance. The sketch opposite epitomises my own struggle to win back 'the soul' and reclaim my pride in being a man.

I have always been struck by the similarities in the freedom fights of disability and blackness. My personal struggle for pride in my disabled identity reflects the larger political struggle of my people towards regaining their self-respect and sense of belonging in their own country. As a young boy in the township, when South Africa was in a 'revolution' and going through its political changes, I was not one of the '76 generation cadres-on-the-front-line. Although I toyi-toyi'd like everyone at the time, I was too young and self-absorbed to be fully involved, sheltered by my family's position from the full impact of the disadvantages and divisions of the past. It was not until my own personal encounter with the 'oppression' of disability that my true political awakening came. I began to look outside myself and to realise the effect of the political inequalities on the lives of people around me. This made me think deeply about the symbolism of being African and the pain that Africa and her people have historically gone through and are still going through. I wrote the following poem in the context of my personal struggle and in the spirit of the African Renaissance. It expresses not only my desire for acceptance as a 'different' man in society, but my feelings about being African. It is my battle cry to regain what was naturally my own, but which was taken away from me as an African and a disabled person – my dignity, my belonging, my beauty, my sense of unity and my pride.

## *I Am What I Am!*

I am an African
The raging beat of a warrior's drum
The rumbling tremor of a Buffalo stampede
The roar of the Lion King in the quiet jungle
I am beauty and pride coated in dark shades
I am gold, diamond and every other precious stone
In the depths of the furrows and the caves is my ancestor's bone
I am the mountains, the running rivers and the trickling streams
I am the rain and the soil, the flower and the bee
From horizon to horizon, coast to coast – all is me

I am a broken African
A sad story of pain, fear and tears narrated by an old man
'I've seen many moons through these wrinkled eyes', he says
I am the horn of a Rhino stolen by a poacher from the other world
The broken wings of an eagle tumbling and drowning in a fall
I am the family swept away by a wave that brought a stranger to my shores
He spoke of love and friendship yet exchanged my beads for chains
Taking with his gushing wave my birth, my land, my flight
I am the songbird singing hoarsely inside a nest of steel bars
The Kingdom and the Heavens razed to ashes in a blaze of change

I am a rising African
The dark cloud that blinds the day, the loud thunder of a brewing storm
I am the burning larva running wild from an exploding volcano – I am war
The river of a nation meandering its dark waters to the raging ocean
A colony of stars that captains a lost vessel out of the deep blue
I am the attempts of a toddler stumbling at the foot of a stairway
The flap of a Phoenix rising from fire, the beauty of a song at dawn
I am the worm that ducks the early-bird, still waters that run deep
I am unity in diversity, from Cape to Cairo I paint the Rainbow
I am an African and proud, from your broken promise I rise reborn

I am a proud African
The stretching blue skies tell the tales of my yesteryear
Unveiling the mysteries of the sacrifice and the bellowing bull
Telling the secrets of the grave and my fears of a hooting owl
The blowing wind whispers the memories of a happier time
When naked children splashed in ponds and frolicked in open fields
And a virgin clutched proudly on a reed, warriors salivating in awe
The crackling lightning screams the story of the nights of light
When wise men passed the calabash, debating family and politics
Falling to their knees at the sight of their King – '*Bayede Ngonyama*!'

*Beka indlebe uzwisise lelolizwi*
'Lend me your ear and listen to the echo of the voices'
*Zwana umzabalazo wesizwe nezinhlupheko*
'Feel the struggle of a nation and its pains'
*Inzukayikeyi nezinswelo nendlala*
'The confusion, the needs and the hunger'
*Kepha kulososicinacina bayahlangana*
'Yet within those confines they come together'
*Wazalwa uNhlangano, yabuya Inkululeko*
'Giving birth to Unity, resurrecting Freedom!'

I am what I am
A nomad that moves his empire with the changing seasons
I am a song of freedom given birth inside the quiet of your dungeons
A single voice of inmates locked away in separate cold cells
The melody of a nightingale spreading its wings to a new-born day
My riches are of beads and skins, gold and diamond, the beauty of my soil
I am a virgin island not fertile and open to alien innuendos
I am the lost Ivory returned to the Tower, pride restored
I am what I am, I sing and dance to the beat of 'I am' and 'I am'
I am an African and so let me be, for that I truly am . . .

I simply am what I am – I am an African!

Scandinavian battlefield mythology tells of Valhalla, a great palace of the gods, where brave warriors slain in war rose anew and gathered together to feast around the great tables, enjoying the victory of everlasting peace. Valhalla was said to be the most mighty palace in Asgard, the realm of the gods. Odin, God of Thunder and War, feasted there with the heroes who were resurrected from the battlefields and brought to the palace by the beautiful Valkyries. The walls of Valhalla were said to be made of gold and the ceiling was formed of gleaming battle shields held up by huge spears. Walls and roof were polished to perfection and their gleam was so bright that it was enough to provide light for the whole palace. The 540 doors were each so wide that 800 men could enter side by side. Odin's guests feasted on long tables and the Valkyries served them with luxurious food and drink. Heroes rode out from there to the battlefield every morning and came back to the palace for noon feasts, where they shared their victories and their wounds were healed.

Fort Valhalla is the name I gave to my house in Pietermaritzburg. This is my 'Hall of Brotherhood', where the warm fires of family togetherness burn day and night. When tragedy struck my life in 1995, it was as if I had been slain and given another chance by life to rise to live again. It was my brothers, more than anyone, who held my hands during that dark time and helped to elevate me from the depths. They made my recovery their personal mission – their own heroic quest. And their steadfastness was what helped me to achieve my healing. It is to them I dedicated the sketch that appears opposite. At the centre of this sketch is a 'Gothic' water jug – representing the sacred life that water bestows. My brothers gave that reviving water to me, and lit the candles of my spirit that had been blown out by the winds of change. Through all the days of darkness that engulfed me, they were there to reassure me of a brighter tomorrow. The edge of the sketch features a bolted frame behind which a hidden dagger signifies the critical moment when death brandished its sword and almost carried me away. My brothers were and always will be my solid ground. They shielded me from pain, danger and further harm – and healed me in the process.

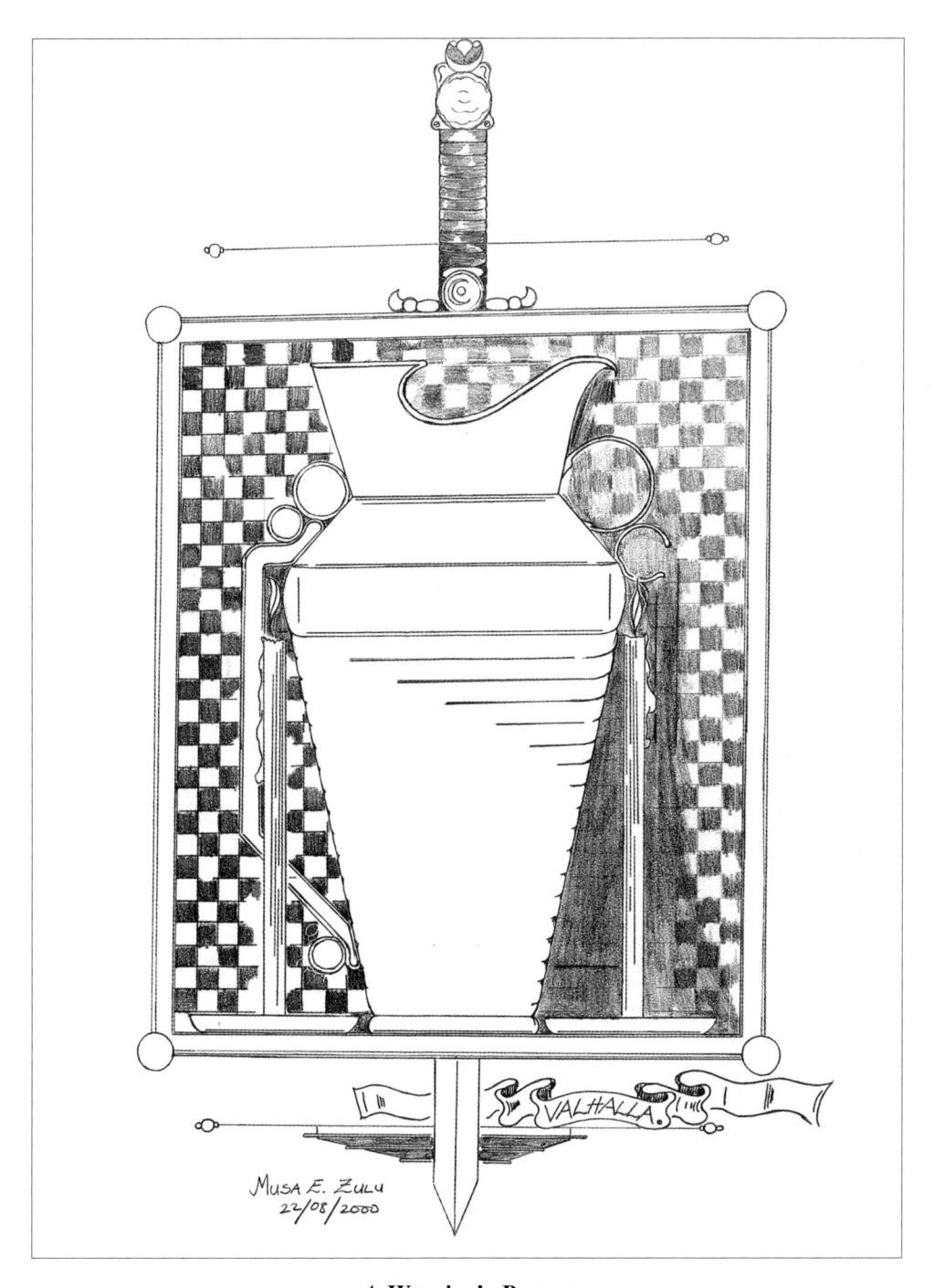

**A Warrior's Prayer**

*Lo there do I see my father. Lo there do I see my mother, my sisters and my brothers. There do I see the line of my people from generations of times long ago. They are calling upon me to take my rightful place – in the Halls of Valhalla – where the brave live forever.*

## *Intimate Selections*

Peace
Childhood fantasies
A young man's dreams
Of space and freedom
Class and style
Light and peace-of-mind

Selective choice reflects
The quest for our sense of belonging
Traces of a place where we want to find a home
Echoes of our need for peace
Selected items – only a few rather than many
An artist's passions mirrored by
His Intimate Selections . . .

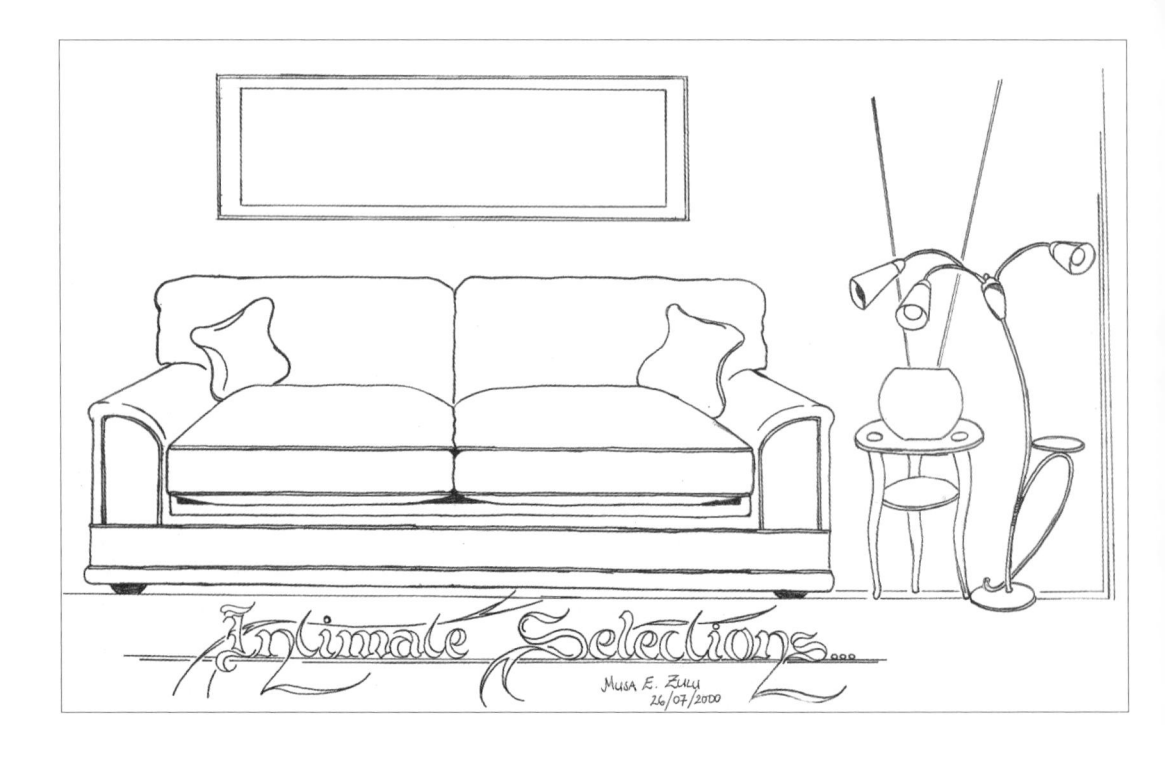

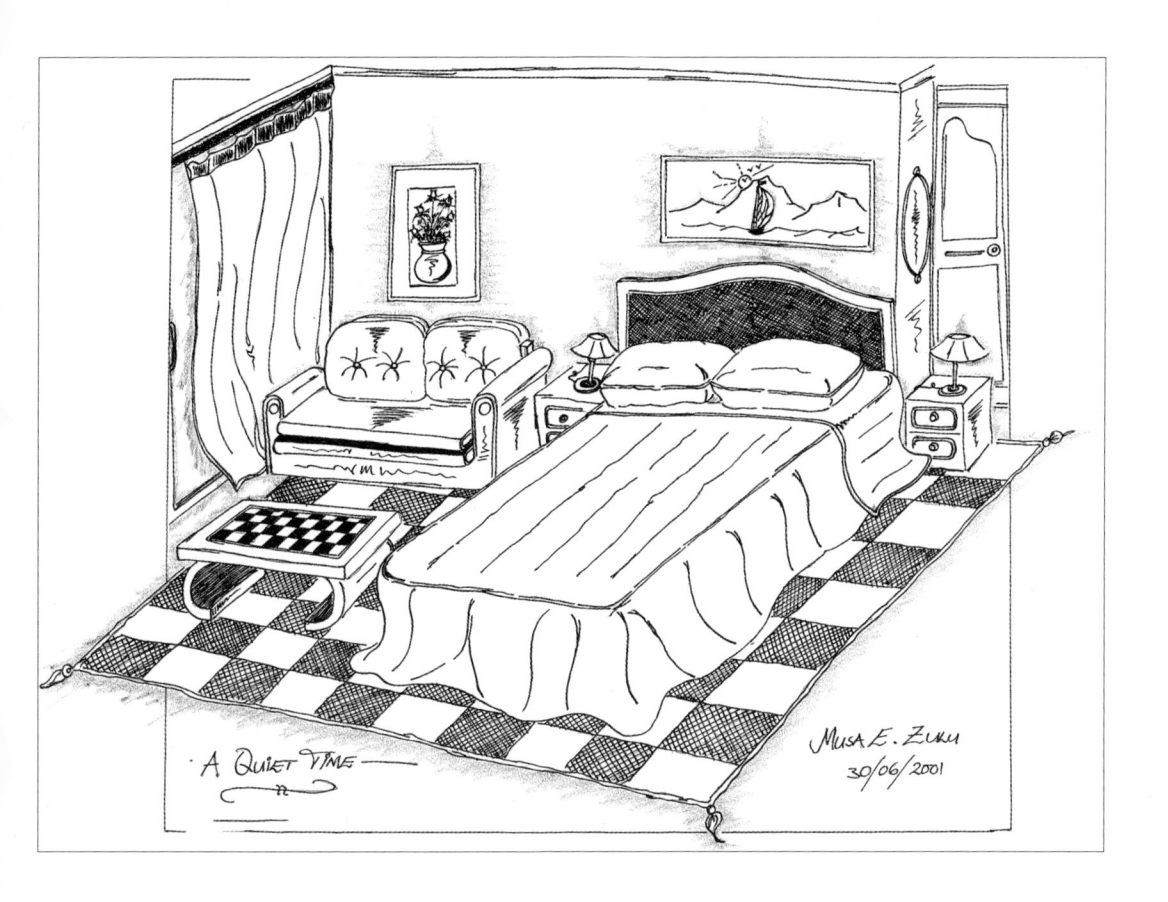

The poem and two drawings opposite and above were done in tribute to my home, Fort Valhalla. It is to Fort Valhalla that I retire at the end of a busy work day, or after long kilometres on the road, to play and unwind and dance to the beat of the favourite old songs. This is where I find time and space to reflect on the changes in my life and write or draw the insights that come to mind. I love my house and have worked hard to make it the haven it is. It reflects my tastes, the 'intimate selections' of my belongings – all the things that I have come to own and cherish. Each of them holds its own meaning and occupies a special place in my heart. The huge couch in the first drawing represents my need for comfort, the light positioned to the right of it, with its branching lamps, is a symbol of the many blessings that have lit my paths in the course of my journey. The little side table stands for the stability and support that my culture and my love of art has provided through all the difficulties. The wall mirror represents my search for answers and solutions that transcend the limitations, and my quest for the best that can be found and experienced. The portrait above is of my bedroom, the sanctuary of 'quiet space' where so much of my creativity happens.

## Last Word

I am . . . one of a kind . . . unique . . . yet part of a unity. Within the small universe of my being is embodied the whole vast miracle of God's creation . . . life and death . . . past, present and future . . . time and eternity. I am just one note in the symphony of life . . . but through me the entire orchestra finds its harmony.

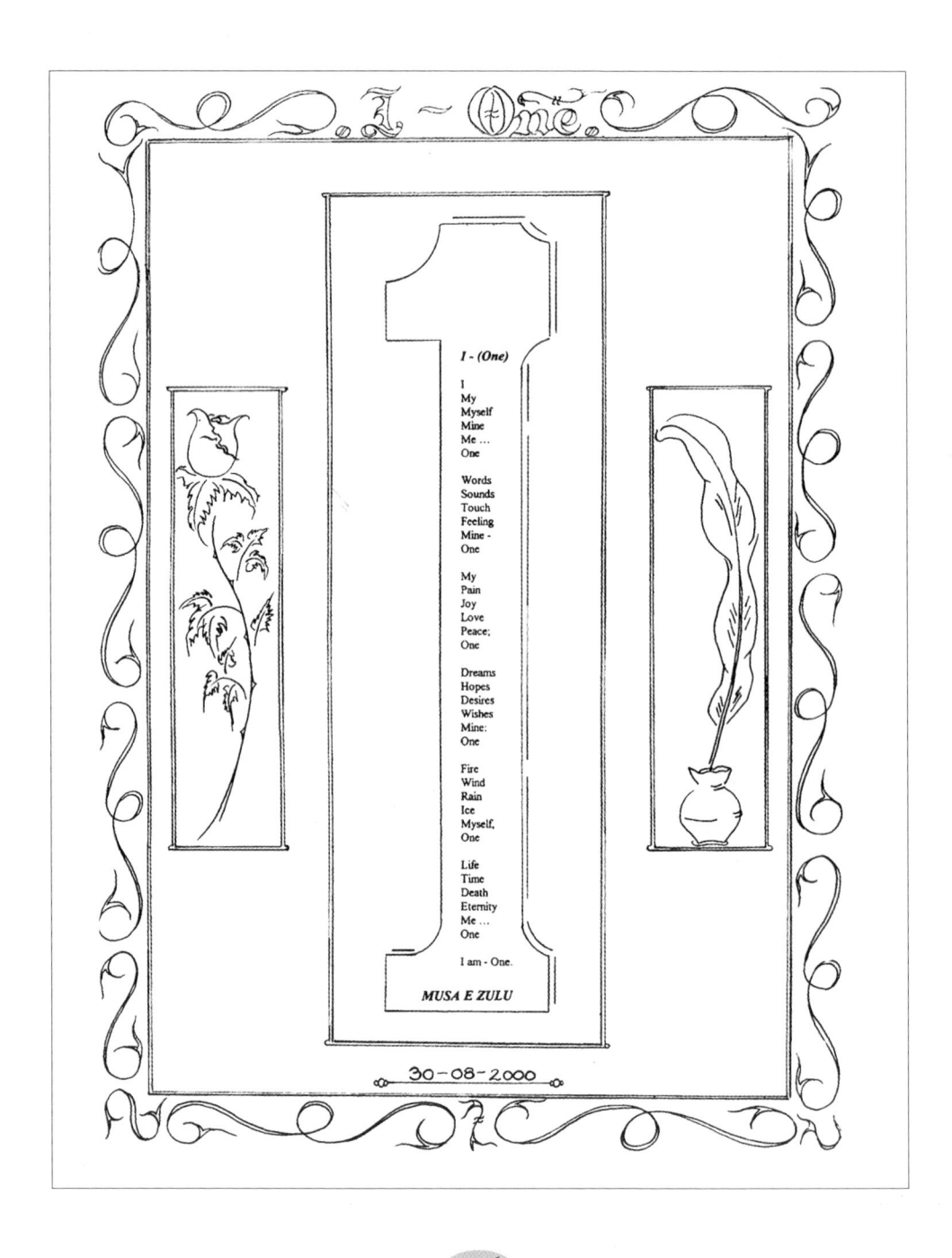

*I ~ One*

### 1 - (One)

I
My
Myself
Mine
Me . . .
One

Words
Sounds
Touch
Feeling
Mine -
One

My
Pain
Joy
Love
Peace;
One

Dreams
Hopes
Desires
Wishes
Mine:
One

Fire
Wind
Rain
Ice
Myself,
One

Life
Time
Death
Eternity
Me . . .
One

I am - One.

**MUSA E ZULU**

30 - 08 - 2000